Principles and Practice of Research in Midwifery

Edited by

Elizabeth R. Cluett MSc SRN SCM PGCEA
Lecturer in Midwifery, School of Nursing and Midwifery,
University of Southampton, Southampton, UK

Rosalind Bluff SRN SCM ADM MTD CertEd(FE) Res Dip
Midwife Teacher and Teaching Fellow, School of Nursing and Midwifery,
University of Southampton, Southampton, UK

Foreword by

Jennifer Sleep BA RN RM MTD
Professor of Nursing and Midwifery Research, Wolfson
Institute of Health Sciences, Thames Valley University,
Reading, UK

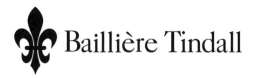

Baillière Tindall

EDINBURGH LONDON NEW YORK OXFORD PHILADELPHIA ST LOUIS SYDNEY TORONTO 2000

BAILLIÈRE TINDALL
An imprint of Elsevier Limited

First published 2000
    Reprinted 2000, 2003, 2004 (twice), 2005

ISBN 0 7020 2425 2

British Library Cataloguing in Publication Data
A catalogue record for this book is available from the British Library

Library of Congress Cataloguing in Publication Data
A catalogue record for this book is available from the Library of Congress

Note
Medical knowledge is constantly changing. As new information becomes available, changes in treatment, procedures, equipment and the use of drugs become necessary. The editors, contributors and the publishers have, as far as it is possible, taken care to ensure that the information given in this text is accurate and up to date. However, readers are strongly advised to confirm that the information, especially with regard to drug usage, complies with the latest legislation and standards of practice.

your source for books, journals and multimedia in the health sciences
www.elsevierhealth.com

Working together to grow
libraries in developing countries
www.elsevier.com | www.bookaid.org | www.sabre.org
ELSEVIER   BOOK AID International   Sabre Foundation

The publisher's policy is to use paper manufactured from sustainable forests

Printed in China
W/07

Contents

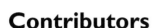

Contributors

Rosalind Bluff SRN SCM ADM MTD CertEd(FE) Res Dip
Midwife Teacher and Teaching Fellow, School of Nursing and Midwifery,
University of Southampton, Southampton, UK

Elizabeth R. Cluett MSc SRN SCM PGCEA
Lecturer in Midwifery, School of Nursing and Midwifery,
University of Southampton, Southampton, UK

Patricia Donovan MA(Ed) MPhil RGN RM ADM PGCEA
Principal Lecturer, University of Central Lancashire, Preston, UK

Ann Robinson MSc RGN RM ADM PGCEA
Clinical Lecturer – Midwifery, European Institute of Health and Medical
Studies, University of Surrey, Guildford, UK

Pam Wagstaff BA(Hons) MSc PGCEA RGN
Lecturer (Neonatal Nursing), School of Nursing and Midwifery,
University of Southampton, Southampton, UK

Foreword

The past two decades have witnessed tremendous developments in midwifery research, both in the number of studies in which midwives have been the lead researchers and also in the quality of the work. Evidence of this can be found in the Midwifery Research Database (MIRIAD) (McCormick & Renfrew 1998), as well as in the growing number of midwife authors who now regularly publish in peer-reviewed journals. This portfolio of studies reflects midwives' willingness to challenge and to provide insights into their own practice, which, in turn, reflects their commitment to providing the highest standards of care for mothers, their babies and their families.

One of the greatest strengths of the research conducted by midwives lies in the rich diversity of methodologies and methods encompassing both naturalist (qualitative) and positivist (quantitative) perspectives. Despite the recent emphasis given to the conduct of randomized trials as the 'gold standard' in relation to evaluation studies, each philosophical approach and each research method has a unique contribution to make to a deeper understanding of practice.

This book is therefore timely in offering an introduction to a whole range of research methods, each of which is given equal consideration. The authors readily acknowledge that although many generic research texts are available, professionals often learn and understand new concepts more easily if they are related to their own individual field of experience. The text thus draws richly on examples specific to maternity care whilst avoiding the pitfalls of separatism, that is, the tendency to consider research conducted by midwives in isolation from the wider aspects of health services research and the global issues of maternal and infant health.

It is good to see that the text is not confined to an exploration of ways of conducting research but also offers an introduction, albeit brief, to evidence-based practice, encompassing the more thorny issues of critical appraisal, dissemination and implementation. In the UK, this is all the more important in the wake of the new DoH requirements concerning Clinical Governance, which place a statutory responsibility upon NHS Trusts, and through them upon health professionals, to demonstrate that clinical decisions are based on sound scientific evidence. Clinicians can no longer choose to ignore research evidence, especially findings which do not equate with their own personal experience and cherished beliefs. Midwives must learn to value ways in which research can inform their practice. A better-informed public will ensure that they do so. With information readily available through an increasing number of multimedia sources including the Internet, the Cochrane Library and MIDIRS information leaflets, midwives need to continue to foster strong and honest partnerships with mothers, families and their local communities. This requires less control, more equality and a willingness to acknowledge the limitations as well as the strengths of current knowledge.

The use of sound research evidence to inform and underpin practice will help to ensure that a woman's remembrance of her childbirth experiences will reflect the very highest standards of midwifery care. A mother never forgets the midwife who delivers her baby.

Jennifer Sleep

REFERENCE

McCormick F, Renfrew M J 1998 The Midwifery Research Database, MIRIAD. A register of information about research in midwifery. Books for Midwives Press, Hale

Acknowledgements

We would like to express our appreciation of the encouragement and support of family, friends and colleagues, without whom this book could not have been written.

1

Introduction

Elizabeth Cluett   Rosalind Bluff

KEY ISSUES

- ◆ History of research in midwifery
- ◆ Definition and purpose of research
- ◆ Evidence-based practice
- ◆ Aim and purpose of book
- ◆ Structure of the book

INTRODUCTION

A midwife is 'able to give the necessary supervision, care and advice to women during pregnancy, labour and the postpartum period, to conduct deliveries on her own responsibility and to care for the newborn and the infant' (UKCC 1998, p. 25).

Every midwife has her own copy of the definition of a midwife, the beginning of which we have chosen to open this book, which explores research from a midwifery perspective. It seems to us that research is implicit within the definition of a midwife. To be able to fulfil the role of the midwife, the practitioner must have the appropriate knowledge base, the skills to provide care and advice as well as the ability to evaluate and update both knowledge and skills. So research must be an integral part of midwifery and therefore the professional life of every midwife. This is endorsed by the report of the Taskforce on the Strategy for Research in Nursing, Midwifery and Health Visiting (Department of Health 1993) which says every practitioner must be 'research literate'.

Throughout this book we have taken 'midwifery' to encompass everything that contributes to the practice of midwifery, and so, while the predominant emphasis is on clinical practice, it also encompasses educational, managerial and professional issues.

HISTORY OF RESEARCH IN MIDWIFERY

Midwifery, in its broadest sense is, as Donnison (1988, p. 11) phrased it 'older than recorded time'. Throughout history midwifery knowledge has developed, changed, been discovered and lost. Yet despite its ancient traditions, or perhaps because of them, research in midwifery, as it is now understood, is very new. Florence Nightingale may have been one of the first to undertake midwifery research. Duff (1998) describes how this renowned nurse's evaluation of maternal mortality in women giving birth in institutions led to some understanding of the dangers of infection and poor hygiene, as independent of poverty and childbirth risks. More recently a key stimulus for research within midwifery was the Briggs Report (Department of Health and Social Security 1972), which advocated that all health professions should be research-based. However, medicine, including obstetrics, already had a long research tradition, with a recognized science-based format since the end of the 18th century, prior to which there was a trial-and-error process of knowledge enhancement. Indeed, the influence of medicine and the scientific tradition in particular has shaped research strategies across all health professions, with nursing and then midwifery drawing on the research knowledge and experience of allied professions.

Midwifery research studies, immediately post-Briggs, seemed to focus on the role of the midwife and the numbers required to provide care (Walker 1976), but some midwives realized the potential of research to contribute to practice and took up the challenge. For example, Jennifer Sleep can be considered a pioneer of midwifery research, having been one of the first to undertake research that was fundamental to midwifery practice. She has also contributed to the support of other midwife researchers, the increase in research awareness and the dissemination of midwifery research. There are many other midwives whose contribution should be recalled, such as Sarah Robinson and Ann Thomson. They contributed to the birth of the Annual Research and the Midwife Conferences, which started in 1978. As research midwives, they recognized the increasing amount of midwifery research being undertaken and wanted both to spread research findings and to encourage other midwives undertaking research projects (Robinson et al 1988). The quality and quantity of midwifery-led research has gone from strength to strength, as testified to by the conferences and their proceedings, and the increasing amount of midwifery research in professional journals. All midwives would be advised to attend conferences where midwifery research is presented. Talking to researchers, hearing how they undertook the studies, the joys and the pitfalls, can enhance understanding of the research process, what it can offer practice and its limitations.

Another key event in the development of midwifery research was the appointment, by the government in 1988, of a midwife researcher, Mary Renfrew, who was based at the National Epidemiology Unit in Oxford (Renfrew 1988). The unit was, and is, renowned for its research into perinatal issues. The appointment of a midwife to the team could be considered as public acknowledgment that midwifery perspectives were unique, could contribute to the wellbeing of women using the maternity service, their families and society, and required the input of midwives. The multidisciplinary nature of the unit meant that research expertise was available and disseminated to others. The profile of midwifery research increased across many organizations associated with maternity care and, significantly, the Midwifery Research Database was born. It could be argued that, despite its short history, midwifery should be a research-aware profession, with several now well-established research information sources. These include the Midwives' Information and Resource Service (MIDIRS) and the Cochrane Collaboration Pregnancy and Childbirth Database. The latter includes systematic reviews, abstracts of reviews of effectiveness, a controlled trials register and a methodology database, which are frequently updated and readily available on computer disk (Cochrane Collaboration 1998). However, research is new to many midwives, and there are always new people entering the profession, and that leads to the aim of this book.

AIM AND PURPOSE OF THE BOOK

There are many research text books available, most relating to medicine or nursing. This book is written predominantly by midwives, for midwives and students of midwifery, although it will be of value to other professionals who have a particular interest in research related to maternity care. Research processes are not unique to midwifery, but we hope to help readers develop a greater understanding of them in a context with which they are already familiar and about which they are knowledgeable. Midwives will be able to envisage the clinical environments that are the research environment and thus come to see how research can be undertaken in a midwifery-related context. Most importantly, midwives will see how research findings can contribute to practice and how they can contribute to the research process.

Hicks (1992) suggested that midwives undervalue research conducted by their peers, and this could be partly due to an inadequate appreciation of research as applied to midwifery. We hope that, if midwives appreciate the quality and breadth of midwifery research, they will not only become increasingly research-aware but value research in midwifery, whether that research was undertaken by midwives or by other professionals with appropriate expertise. Research has a strong science and medical influence; these are traditionally male domains and Rodgers (1986) suggests that this gives research the image of being a masculine subject. Thus the initial poor uptake of research by midwives, and the undervaluing of midwifery research by other midwives, could be a gender issue, which we hope to dispel.

Meah et al (1996) suggested that one barrier to greater use of research findings by midwives was their lack of confidence in evaluating findings and deciding if they should be incorporated into their practice. We hope that this book makes research more accessible to midwives, with the ultimate aim of improving the care offered to women and their families, by enhancing access to, and understanding and appropriate use of, the latest research findings. Some fear that research, like statistics, can be manipulated to say what authors want. While to a degree this is true, the ability to understand and critique research reports should give midwives the confidence to read such papers, using an evaluation framework to help them determine their worth, rather than denigrating all research through fear and/or ignorance.

We have suggested that midwives need to be research-aware. Research awareness has been well described by Clark (1987) and, although applied to nurses, the understanding of 'research awareness' is equally valid for midwives. We consider that being 'research-aware' means being able to:

◆ identify areas that might benefit from research in your own practice
◆ identify areas in service provision that might benefit from research
◆ identify new ideas or technologies that need to be investigated
◆ read published papers pertaining to practice and evaluate their suitability for implementation
◆ seek out literature on any subject to meet the needs of a client or client group
◆ make research findings available in a user-friendly form as part of parent education activities
◆ help others understand the strengths and weaknesses of research findings
◆ advise and support women who are asked to participate in research
◆ support midwives undertaking research
◆ evaluate whether the research you are being asked to collect data for is being properly conducted and is in the best interests of the participants.

This list may not be complete but it does demonstrate that being research-aware involves a broad range of knowledge and skills. These are not 'once and for all' skills, but an ongoing process of acquiring and using knowledge to steadily deepen your research understanding. This book recognizes that individual midwives will be at various stages of research awareness and aims to help consolidate and increase that awareness.

DEFINITION AND PURPOSE OF RESEARCH

Having identified that all midwives need to be research-aware, and that it is integral to midwifery practice, it is necessary to consider what research is, and its relationship to other forms of literature.

There are many definitions of research. The most basic meaning is 'to examine carefully' (Burns and Grove 1993, p. 3), but most definitions are expanded to include some explanation as well as a definition, for example:

◆ 'an attempt to increase available knowledge by the discovery of new facts or relationships through a process of systematic scientific enquiry' (Macleod Clark and Hockey 1996, p. 4)
◆ 'systematic inquiry that uses orderly scientific methods to answer questions or solve problems' (Polit and Hungler 1997, p. 467)
◆ 'rigorous and systematic inquiry conducted on a scale and using methods commensurate with the issue investigated, and designed to lead to contributions to generalizable knowledge' (Department of Health 1993, p. 6).

These are only a few definitions but they share a common meaning, that of gaining knowledge via a planned strategy. However they do not fully define research, for research is not merely about discovering facts, it is also about exploring the relationships between facts and confirming the facts in relation to a variety of situations and people at various times. So it is useful to consider the purpose of research in relation to midwifery practice and the provision of maternity care, rather than just a definition of research. The one overriding purpose must be to improve the outcomes and experiences of childbirth for all involved in the process. This global aim can be divided into a series of interrelated aims, although these have been, and are, equally applicable to many other spheres of life, not just midwifery:

◆ to gain an ever-deepening understanding of the physiological, psychological and sociological aspects of the childbearing process
◆ to develop a sound rationale for midwifery practice
◆ to increase the variety of options available to those involved in the childbearing process
◆ to develop standards of care and thus contribute to quality assurance
◆ to contribute to the provision of cost-effective care.

This list could be extended: for example, Hockey (1996) presented aims for nursing research that included establishing and enhancing multidisciplinary and international relationships, which would then enhance care. Hockey (1996) also suggested that the improvement of the professional status of nursing was an aim of nursing research. While high-quality research may result in the enhancement of a particular professional group, the key purpose of health-care research should be the improvement of the wellbeing of the target group, with any additional benefits being fortuitous. The history of midwifery research tends to confirm that its primary aim is that of enhancing the quality and provision of care. It could also be argued that, if midwifery practitioners wish to be advocates for high-quality, woman-centred care, they must be able to do so from a position of equality with other professional groups. Achieving professional academic and practice status by demonstrating a researched knowledge base may therefore indirectly improve midwifery care.

The discussion above seems to indicate that research is the answer to all midwifery problems. Unfortunately, it is not. There will never be enough research undertaken to answer the question: What do we do in this situation for this woman? The best we can hope for is that research findings will be available as guidance for the most common events; they will never be specific to individual women. So research information must be seen within the context of the wider information pool, which includes clinical audits, traditional practice and personal experiences, all of which are disseminated via personal contact and through journals and textbooks in the form of reports, editorials, reviews and letters. They may originate from governments, professional organizations, experts or individual practitioners. Each has a valid contribution to make, but it is the responsibility of the practitioner to evaluate each source, its quality and whether or not it should influence practice.

Research and audit are two processes that have some similarities, as both may use the same data collection methods and tools, which can lead to confusion. Research can be considered as a process aiming to discover or confirm new information, while audit assesses whether resources are being appropriately used in practice and reflects the knowledge and standards already established (Crombie et al 1993, Hundley and Graham 1997). In this way, audit and research compliment each other. High-quality research and clinical audit combined are cornerstones of clinical governance, which together contribute to a high-quality and effective maternity service, now a requirement of all NHS services (Department of Health 1998). This book does not focus on audit, which is often linked to assessing the quality of a service and for which other texts are available (Buckley 1997); however, participation in an audit may be a midwife's first introduction to data collection and analysis. Methods used in audit may overlap with those used in quantitative research, particularly survey-type studies, which use similar tools – such as questionnaires and both descriptive and correlational statistics, which are discussed in later chapters.

EVIDENCE-BASED PRACTICE

So far, we have emphasized that midwifery should be a research-based profession. However, as already intimated, research findings may not be available, and thus something further is needed: this is the concept of evidence-based practice. Evidence-based practice has been well described by Sackett et al (1997, p. 71), who define it as 'the conscientious, explicit and judicious use of current best evidence in making decisions about the care of individual patients'.

This is more than just research-based practice. Evidence-based practice recognizes the value of experience, of professional sensitivity and inter-personal dynamics between women and their carers. Gray (1997) suggests that evidence-based practice means including the client within the decision-making process, a philosophy that is commensurate with a partnership between the woman and midwife. To be an evidence-based practitioner means not just knowing the research terminology and the latest research findings, and indiscriminately applying them in practice, but integrating them in a holistic way to meet the needs of women. It is the unique and almost endless ways in which knowledge and skills are integrated to meet the needs of individual women within their milieu that can be considered the craft of midwifery (Magill-Cuerden 1993). So, having considered the science of research, we now can explore the art of applying research findings to practice. Just as it is not the colours used by a painter that make him great, but how those colours are used, so knowledge and skills alone cannot make good midwives: the art is in how they use that knowledge and skills in their care of women. As Page (1997) suggests, evidence-based practice equates very well to the art and science of midwifery. For the midwife, this means having an important combination of skills and characteristics, which include being:

◆ observant and sensitive and thus able to identify the needs of individual women
◆ empathic to the needs women may not be able to articulate
◆ an effective communicator, to enable women to be equal partners in their care
◆ a reflective practitioner, and therefore able to develop clinical expertise based on personal practice and experience
◆ questioning and open to questions in all aspects of practice
◆ a lifelong learner – knowledge is never stationary and the midwife must continuously and conscientiously keep her/himself updated
◆ research-aware.

This combination of characteristics will enable the midwife to use research evidence effectively *and* judiciously apply it to the needs of the individual. The aim of this book is to contribute to the development and enhancement of the last characteristic in the above list and thus assist the midwife to practise evidence-based midwifery. However this is not a one-off achievement:

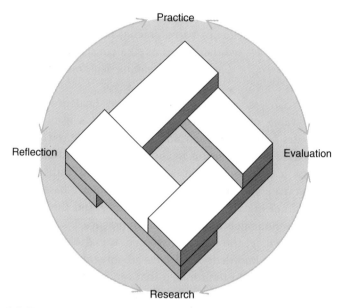

Figure 1.1 The never-ending steps of research: a representation of research and midwifery to achieve evidence-based practice

evidence-based practice could be likened to the impossible staircase, always going up (Fig. 1.1).

At two of the four corners are reflection and evaluation, as both these processes are essential for quality practice and research. The upwards spiral highlights that there is no end to this process: this is the principle of lifelong learning. The two-way arrows indicate that all the key points are interchangeable and equally vital. With this concept in mind we invite you to read the rest of the book.

STRUCTURE OF THE BOOK

The chapters in this book are written by practitioners who all have a maternal or neonatal focus, a clinical background and experience in the research approach on which they write. This has resulted in each chapter adopting a different writing style, although the overall structure remains constant throughout. The book can be read in its entirety, but each chapter can be consulted independently.

Chapter 2 provides the foundation for all subsequent chapters by considering the nature of midwifery practice, then exploring the nature of knowledge and theory. This leads on to the consideration of the main philosophies under-pinning research, and hence quantitative and qualitative research. The relationship between midwifery and these approaches, as well as the relationship between the approaches themselves, is considered. In this introductory chapter we have indicated that research is integral to midwifery, and this is an ongoing theme of the book. Therefore, Chapter 2 concludes by considering how research originates from practice, which is the starting point of every research study.

Chapters 3–8 each focus on one approach to research and consider the nature of that approach, its origins, and the methods and tools that may be used. Advantages and disadvantages and, where appropriate, the practicalities of the research methods are discussed. Chapter 9 takes a broader perspective, looking at a variety of other research approaches. Examples of midwifery research are used to illustrate the issues under discussion.

It is only possible to critique a research paper once you have some understanding of the research approaches, methods and tools involved (Parahoo 1997). Therefore, Chapter 10 builds on the information that has been provided throughout previous chapters and considers a framework with key elements for consideration when critiquing research articles/papers. The emphasis throughout has been on understanding research to enhance practice and so the final chapter takes the research findings/knowledge back into practice and completes the circle by emphasizing the practice–research link.

Throughout the book, please look out for new and less familiar research terms, which are printed in bold type when introduced. These words are all defined in the glossary at the end of the book.

REFERENCES

Buckley, E R 1997 Delivering quality in midwifery. Baillière Tindall, London

Burns N, Grove S K 1993 The practice of nursing research. Conduct, critique and utilization, 2nd edn. WB Saunders, Philadelphia, PA

Clark E 1987 Research awareness: its importance in practice. Professional Nurse 2(11): 371–373

Cochrane Collaboration 1998 The Cochrane Library. Cochrane Collaboration and Software Ltd, Oxford

Crombie I K, Davies H T O, Abraham S C S, Florey C 1993 The audit handbook. Improving health care through clinical audit. John Wiley, Chichester

Department of Health 1993 Report of the Taskforce on the Strategy for Research in Nursing, Midwifery and Health Visiting. HMSO, London

Department of Health 1998 NHS to have legal duty of ensuring quality for the first time (Press Release 98/141, 13th April). HMSO, London

Department of Health and Social Security 1972 Report of the Committee into Nursing. (The Briggs Report.) HMSO, London

Donnison J 1988 Midwives and medical men. A history of the struggle for the control of childbirth. Historical Publication, London

Duff E 1998 Florence Nightingale: basing care on evidence. RCM Midwives Journal 1(6): 192–193

Gray M J A 1997 Evidence-based healthcare: how to make health policy and management decisions. Churchill Livingstone, Edinburgh

Hicks C M 1992 Research in midwifery: are midwives their own worst enemies? Midwifery 8(1): 12–18

Hockey L 1996 The nature and purpose of research. In: Cormack D F S (ed) The research process in nursing, 3rd edn. Blackwell Science, Oxford, ch 1, p 3–13

Hundley V, Graham W 1997 Research and audit in midwifery: does the difference matter? British Journal of Midwifery 5(11): 664–668

Macleod Clark J, Hockey L 1996 The relevance of research to nursing. In: Macleod Clark J, Hockey L (ed) Further research for nursing. A new guide for the enquiring nurse. Scutari Press, London, ch 1, p 3–11

Magill-Cuerden J 1993 Midwifery is an old craft and a new science. In: International Confederation of Midwives 23rd International Congress, Vancouver, Canada. Proceedings, vol 2, p 1152–1165

Meah S, Luker K A, Cullum N A 1996 An exploration of midwives' attitudes to research and perceived barriers to research utilization. Midwifery 12(1): 73–84

Page L 1997 Evidence based maternity care: science and sensitivity in practice. New Generation Digest Dec 20: 2–3

Parahoo A K 1997 Nursing research. Principles, process and issues. Macmillan, Basingstoke

Polit D F, Hungler B P 1997 Essentials of nursing research. Methods, appraisal and utilization, 4th edn. JB Lippincott, Philadelphia, PA

Renfrew M 1988 Developing midwifery research: the role of the midwife researcher at the national perinatal epidemiology unit. Research and the Midwife Conference Proceedings: 86–89

Robinson S, Thomson A, Ticker V 1988 Midwives' views on directions and development in midwifery research. Research and the Midwife Conference Proceedings: 90–103

Rodgers C 1986 Sex roles in education. In: Hargreaves D J, Colley A M (ed) The psychology of sex rules. Harper & Row, London

Sackett D L, Richardson W S, Rosenberg W, Haynes R B 1997 Evidence-based medicine. How to practise and teach EBM. Churchill Livingstone, Edinburgh

UKCC 1998 Midwives' rules and code of practice. United Kingdom Central Council for Nursing, Midwifery and Health Visiting, London

Walker J 1976 Midwife or obstetric nurse? Some perceptions of midwives and obstetricians of the role of the midwife. Journal of Advanced Nursing 1: 129–138

2

From practice to research

Elizabeth Cluett   Rosalind Bluff

KEY ISSUES

- ◆ Portrait of midwifery and the need for research
- ◆ Theory
- ◆ From practice to research
- ◆ Types of knowledge
- ◆ What is research?

INTRODUCTION

The aim of this chapter is to consider practice, and show how research can be derived from the clinical domain and what the role of the midwife is in facilitating that process. One type of research could never reflect the many facets of midwifery, and therefore a variety of research approaches are required. This introduces a philosophy that suggests that all research methods can be equally valid within midwifery. An individual research approach cannot be right or wrong (this is not to say that it cannot be incorrectly undertaken, which is a different issue); however, for a given project, one approach may be more appropriate than another. As every research study is embedded within a knowledge base and within a philosophy, this chapter will begin by exploring the important concepts that underpin the rest of the book. These concepts are midwifery practice, knowledge, theory and research.

A PORTRAIT OF MIDWIFERY – IS RESEARCH NEEDED?

To explore how research develops from midwifery practice it is first necessary to consider the question: What is midwifery practice? There are as many answers to this question as there are midwives and women who have been cared for by midwives. There is a well-recognized definition of a midwife and a list of the midwife's activities in the Midwives' Code of Practice (UKCC 1998), but midwifery is far broader than any definition or list of activities. Bryar (1995) suggests that 'to be a midwife is to use the self': in other words, the personality of the individual midwife cannot be separated from her/his midwifery practice. But midwifery practice must be broader than any individual or group of individuals. A view of midwifery practice and how it has evolved over time can be obtained from Donnison 1988, Towler and Bramall 1986 and by considering how midwifery and the role of the midwife is portrayed through the many editions of midwifery texts such as *Mayes' Midwifery* (current edition, Sweet 1997) or Myles' *Textbook for Midwives* (current edition, Bennett and Brown 1993). You could also consider the changing attitude of governments to the maternity services and midwifery, highlighted in the *Changing Childbirth Report* (Department of Health 1993) and the Standing Nursing and Midwifery Advisory Committee (SNMAC) Report, *Midwifery: Delivering our Future* (Department of Health 1998). The social and cultural climate of the times, as well as medical and technological advances, greatly influence midwifery practice, both in what society wants from midwifery and what midwifery is able to offer. It could be argued that the only way to really get a portrait of midwifery is to experience midwifery, but how? As a consumer, a midwife, a health visitor, a general practitioner, an obstetrician, an obstetric physiotherapist, the list is endless. Perhaps the way to gain the 'midwifery picture' is to explore, describe and catalogue it, but what would be explored:

◆ the number of women delivered normally
◆ the number of antepartum/intrapartum/postpartum events
◆ the number of hours worked by midwives
◆ what contributes to a normal delivery
◆ the satisfaction of women/their partners/midwives
◆ the size and types of maternity units, including the decor inside
◆ expectations and experiences of women and their families
◆ the quantity of thank-you letters or complaints
◆ the uptake of midwifery-led care as opposed to obstetric-led care
◆ the amount of postnatal depression/postpartum traumatic stress disorder
◆ the percentage of health-care funding allocated to midwifery
◆ the amount of research related to midwifery?

The above list is only a beginning: every woman and midwife could add to it, but it clearly shows that midwifery is complex and multifaceted. In addition, midwifery is dynamic. Whereas the main priority was once a live mother and baby, in a culture where this is the norm the emphasis has changed to include a fulfilling birth experience where the woman has choices and control of the care she receives (Department of Health 1993). The midwife has changed too – many are educated through diploma and degree programmes with expectations that they will be autonomous practitioners and function within a multidisciplinary health-care team. There is currently emphasis on practitioners to be 'fit for the purpose', with the 'competencies' (Phillips et al 1994, Fraser et al 1997) required for modern practice but midwives must also be 'sensitive' (Flint 1986, Page 1997) so each woman feels special. Therefore the only way to understand such a complex phenomenon as midwifery is through careful exploration of its many facets. This can only be achieved through meticulous attention to detail, documentation of events, identifying interdependent components, by understanding what midwifery means to the individuals and groups who come into contact with midwifery, looking for relationships, including causal links, between the various events that contribute to midwifery care, and by considering all the evidence as to what is or could be midwifery. This is the scope of midwifery research and for high-quality practice it is essential.

TYPES OF KNOWLEDGE

One aim of research is to advance the knowledge on which midwifery practice is built, which includes not merely extending knowledge boundaries but consolidating and confirming them. Indeed, if midwives are to be autonomous practitioners they need to be able to justify their practice, to women, society and other professionals, articulating the knowledge underpinning their activities. As knowledge and research are inextricably linked it is essential to consider the nature of knowledge. The study of the nature of knowledge is called **epistemology**, and is a field in its own right. Here we will only present a brief overview of the different types of knowledge as we feel they contribute to the understanding of research within midwifery practice.

Traditional knowledge

Much of midwifery practice is based on tradition (Department of Health 1993, Hurley 1998), i.e. practice based on beliefs handed down from one generation to the next. Practice becomes an established custom or part of the culture and can become routine or ritualistic. For example, measuring the height of the postpartum uterine fundus as an evaluation of involution can be traced to 1895 (Cluett et al 1995). Practice based on tradition may not reflect the best evidence currently available and, when challenged, the response from some midwives is 'this is the way we've always done it' (Bluff, ongoing study). It is acknowledged by midwives, students and women (Department of Health 1993) that practice based on this type of knowledge does not meet women's needs, resulting in care that is less than optimal. It is important to remember that, when there is no evidence to inform practice, it will continue to be based on tradition (Jackson 1994), and that may be appropriate. It is, however, no longer acceptable to introduce new practices without evaluation, otherwise new traditions are generated.

Common sense

Jackson (1994) believes that midwifery practice is often based on common sense. Clark (1987) suggests that 'common' implies something that is taken for granted and is widely accepted and agreed upon, while 'sense' suggests some type of reasoning. This does appear to be a contradiction in terms. 'Taken for granted' does not mean that thought has been given to the topic. As common sense may be based on values and beliefs, this can be a form of traditional knowledge. Conversely, because midwives practise in different environments and cultures, what is common sense to one practitioner may not be to another.

Trial and error

If there is a lack of knowledge of what care to provide, decisions may be made through trial and error. If one form of care is unsatisfactory then another is adopted until a solution is identified. In this way, knowledge is gained through clinical experience. While this may be safe, if all the options tried have previously been tested, the invention of a new option may expose women and their infants to unknown dangers. In addition, this is not a useful means of gaining knowledge as the process has to be repeated with each client because you never know which option will have the desired effect. This is not to exclude new ideas, but they cannot be thoughtlessly introduced.

Intuitive knowledge

Benner (1984) recognizes that knowledge is embedded in practice. Expert practitioners act on intuition. Polanyi (1958) and Benner (1984) refer to intuition as tacit knowledge, meaning something we know but cannot articulate. This may consist of knowledge that we have gained in the classroom or from clinical experience, or a composite of many learning opportunities. It is the recognition of tacit knowledge that has contributed to the increased emphasis on reflection on practice (Schön 1983, Boud et al 1985), which aims to help individuals make this knowledge explicit and thus open to expression, debate and transmission to others. Paul and Heaslip (1995) argue that, when practice is based on intuitive knowledge to which we give no thought, or where we think we have more knowledge than we actually have, it can lead to inaccurate judgements that could adversely affect the quality of care we provide. When intuition is combined with critical thinking and reflection to help us identify what we do and do not know, we then avoid inappropriate decisions (Paul and Heaslip 1995). The key then is to remain alert and questioning of our practice.

Experience

Knowledge that is gained from clinical experience is important to midwives (Mander 1992). While such knowledge is valuable it is important to remember that it can become out of date. The experience of the midwife may be limited because she/he has recently qualified or has worked within a restricted setting or client group. Neither can it be isolated from life experiences, communication and organizational skills, as well as skills gained through personal loss and crisis, to mention but a few. All contribute to knowledge that is drawn upon in practice and this links directly with personal knowledge.

Personal knowledge

Polanyi (1958) adopts a broad view of personal knowledge, while Carper (1978) relates such knowledge to knowing the self or being self-aware, which fits well with Bryar's (1995) concept of the midwife being 'inextricable' from the individual person. It is with this knowledge that midwives can develop therapeutic relationships with their clients. Through knowing the self, we can be conscious of how we behave and the effects we have on each other and those we care for. Self-awareness is also the means by which we can be authentic; however, some midwives lack this personal knowledge (Bluff, ongoing study).

THEORY

Just as an understanding of the types of knowledge contributes to an overall understanding of research in its widest application and aims, there needs to be some understanding of what is meant by theory. Indeed, it could be argued that all research is theory-dependent. There is either a theory that the research aims to test and/or quantify, as in many quantitative studies, or there is an idea that there is an unknown theory, which the researcher is trying to elucidate, as in most qualitative studies.

Bryar (1995, p. 2) states that 'frequent comments are made about the lack of theory in midwifery', without identifying the source of these comments. Whatever the source, the impression may be due to a lack of understanding of the concept of a 'theory'. As Bryar (1995) points out, midwives integrate knowledge and skills to provide care, which implies a degree of theory that underpins practice. Gilbert (1993) suggests that theory is the proposed explanation for any given situation, which concurs with Bryar (1995, p. 28), who says that theory 'is essentially about providing explanations of events, actions and phenomena'. These explanations are formed when concepts are linked together, where a concept is an idea or abstract thought, derived from knowledge, that enables us to make sense of what is happening around us and therefore guides our practice. But, as Bryar (1995) and others (Chinn and Kramer 1991, Perry 1997) acknowledge, the issue of theory is a complex one. Numerous definitions exist and those wishing to consider the nature of theory further are advised to refer to other texts, including those cited above. It is important to remember that there may be more than one theory to explain a phenomenon, and this may in part account for variations in practice.

It could be argued that knowledge unique to midwifery provides theory of midwifery while knowledge from other disciplines that is applied to midwifery provides additional theory for practice. This would include knowledge from biohealth, sociology, psychology, medicine, mental health and many other disciplines. It is the way such knowledge is integrated that makes it midwifery theory, which could therefore be defined as all the knowledge midwives use to inform their practice. If we use Bryar's (1995) understanding of theory it becomes apparent that there is no lack of theory in relation to midwifery practice. Midwives use the types of knowledge we have so far considered to develop their own theories based on observation, experience and reflection. These aim to explain what happens in midwifery settings and the care given to women. The disadvantage of such theories is that, although there is often a lack of evidence to support their use, we have no alternative but to rely on them to inform our practice. Theories are dynamic: as new knowledge emerges, theories may be rejected or modified and new theories developed. For this reason it is imperative that midwives update themselves in order to provide quality care. Sometimes we may lack the knowledge necessary to develop a theory. In the absence of such knowledge there is the tendency to make assumptions. It is from these assumptions that stereotypes are formed. Care given by midwives may be adversely influenced when it is based on stereotypes.

WHAT IS RESEARCH?

So far we have considered types of knowledge and what theory is, and could conclude that practice is the utilization of theories by midwives based on knowledge from a variety of sources, which may or may not be validated. In its broadest sense, research is a process that strives to increase and validate knowledge, thus contributing to the provision of evidence on which to base midwifery theories and practice. This is achieved by either testing theory or generating theory. We will now consider theory testing and theory generating as the main broad approaches to research.

Where there is a suggested theory, research aims to test the presence, strength and inter-relationships of that theory. This is a **deductive** research process: the theory is expressed and steps are taken to either accept or reject the proposed theory. When there is no proposed theory an **inductive** process is adopted, which aims to identify and develop the underlying theory through detailed description and analysis of the situation.

Every theory must have come from somewhere. Usually, it has arisen from an observed event. A midwife may have noticed that women who have had a child before deliver more quickly than those who have not. The proposed theory would be:

second and subsequent births are shorter than the first,

which could then be tested by comparing a number of first and subsequent births. This may be called a **hypothetico-deductive** process. A hypothetical theory has been proposed, which can then be tested. If the theory is rejected, an alternative one is suggested, which is tested. If the original theory is accepted, then theories as to why it is so are suggested and tested, and so on in a forward-spiralling process. This deductive approach has been traditionally associated with hard science, where the research testing has been undertaken within a laboratory-type setting or a controlled situation. This is also referred to as the positivist tradition, as the emphasis is on 'positive science' (Kaplan 1968, cited in Parahoo 1997). Here the philosophy is that 'the truth is out there' (apologies to *The X Files*) – that facts are objective and can therefore be identified and measured. This is the biomedical stance, with traditions based in chemistry, physics and biology, and is recognized as the research model adopted by the medical professions. This is the **quantitative** approach to research.

Inductive research has developed from a **humanistic** approach. Here a question is identified,

Is the experience different for women if they are having their first or second baby?

Having posed the question (qualitative researchers may prefer to consider a statement indicating the area of focus rather than a question), information is collected in order to answer it. The information is used to describe the situation, then classify it in some order, to give meaning to the answer, and so a theory may be developed. The humanistic approach is attributed mostly to the social sciences, and as a result takes a more personal perspective – that truth is determined by the person within the situation, or is context-specific. This is subjective, but it could be argued that it is an honest approach. This is equated to a **qualitative** approach to research, where qualitative research is primarily concerned with explaining, interpreting and understanding how people see their world. Each person's view of the world is different and therefore there are multiple realities. It could be argued that this reflects the caring, woman-centred, philosophy of midwifery.

By now you may well think that inductive and deductive approaches are actually two sides of the same coin, i.e. different perspectives of the same process, and to some extent you would be right. Indeed Gilbert (1993), who uses diagrams to depict the relationship between practice (which he refers to as the social world), data and theory for inductive and deductive processes, acknowledges that, although the two approaches are by definition separate, in practice they overlap. These two main research approaches are often called research paradigms, where **paradigm** means taking a particular perspective or point of view. Kuhn (1970), to whom is attributed the first use of the term paradigm (Parahoo 1997), used it to mean a specific school of thought, which has since been developed to encompass all the beliefs and assumptions associated with one perspective or stance. There are generally considered to be two main perspectives or viewpoints, the **positivist** and the **interpretist**, also referred to as the quantitative and qualitative research paradigms. We believe that they are not completely independent, but complementary, with the same aim, that of increasing knowledge in relation to midwifery practice. One way of expressing the relationship between the two paradigms is to use a continuum, where there can be progression in either direction (Fig. 2.1).

This continuum is not complete: other research approaches could be included and there is scope for new ones to be added as they are developed.

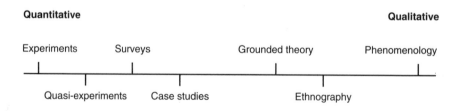

Note: spacing is for ease of reading and is not significant.

Figure 2.1 A research continuum

PARADIGMS, APPROACHES, METHODOLOGY AND METHODS: A TERMINOLOGY DEBATE

So far, we have referred to the two main research paradigms or perspectives, the quantitative and the qualitative paradigms. Within each paradigm there are several research approaches where an approach can be considered a type of research. For example, experimental and survey approaches are within the quantitative paradigm while grounded theory and ethnography fall within the qualitative paradigm.

Methodology is another term frequently used. Sidell (1989, p. 261) defined methodology as 'the theoretical assumptions upon which the choice of a particular research method is based'. This could be equated to either the paradigm or the approach adopted for a study, or both. Methodology is often confused with **method**, which is the specific tools and techniques used to conduct a particular study. So a questionnaire could be the selected method and could be appropriate for several research approaches. Often, several different tools or methods are used in one study; the combination of these is the research **design**. The research design is the detailed plan of how the research was conducted and from it other researchers should be able to duplicate the process. The design may be unique to a study but, particularly in quantitative research approaches, the designs may be well established, such as the randomized controlled trial, which will be considered in Chapter 3. This has led to the term 'design' being used interchangeably with 'method' by some.

There are alternative meanings for other key research terms. For example, Reid (1993) and Cormack (1996) use the term 'approach' to refer to the two paradigms (i.e. quantitative or qualitative). Mulhall (1994) seems to use the terms approach and design synonymously, with approach being related to qualitative research and designs to quantitative research. Polit and Hungler (1997) refer to a methodological distinction between quantitative and qualitative research, which seems to equate 'methodology' with 'approach', but they then go on to refer to scientific and naturalistic methods. Hicks (1996) uses 'approach' in relation to the type of statistics used. The conclusion must be that different authors use research terms differently, and with slightly different meanings in various contexts. We can only advise that you try and identify the key research terms in the text and establish how they are being used in that context (Box 2.1).

This classification is rather rigid and, while it is intended to be of assistance, it will become evident as you read through the chapters that it is impossible to completely divide one approach from another or one method or design from another. Where approaches are blurred this is called **method slurring**. It is the modification of one approach or method to meet the needs of a specific research study or clinical setting. This is acceptable: just as midwives aim to

> **Box 2.1** Summary of research terms adopted throughout this book
>
> ◆ **Paradigm:** the perspective or viewpoint adopted, quantitative or qualitative
> ◆ **Approach:** the types of research within the perspectives – experimental/ethnography
> ◆ **Method:** the tools and techniques used to undertake the study
> ◆ **Design:** the research plan, what is done and when

provide individualized care, modifying various care options to meet the needs of the woman, so researchers may need to modify the research process. As in practice, it is vital that all modifications are clearly identified and documented, and that careful consideration is given to the effects of the modifications on the research process and findings.

THE MAIN ASSUMPTIONS FOR EACH RESEARCH APPROACH

We have already identified the background to the qualitative and quantitative research paradigms, but there are several other features that are associated with each approach, which in turn helps identify the types of research method that each approach most commonly adopts. These features are compared in Table 2.1.

Table 2.1 The main features of the quantitative and qualitative approaches to research

Quantitative research	Qualitative research
Deductive	Inductive
Positivist	Humanistic
Facts as independent	Facts as context-dependent
Aims to be objective	Recognizes subjectivity
Tests a hypothesis	Answers a question or fulfils an aim
Experimental to survey experimental approaches (designs)	Grounded theory to phenomenological approaches
Statistical analysis predominant	Analysis of words

There has been a tendency to assume that deductive or quantitative research is superior to inductive or qualitative research. This may have more to do with traditional power and gender issues associated with the sciences than with the actual value of the approaches. In this text quantitative and qualitative research are both considered to have strengths and weaknesses that may make them more suitable for some scenarios than others, but both have a useful contribution to make to developing a greater understanding of midwifery practice. This imbalance is ongoing, with the randomized controlled trial, the classical quantitative method, being considered to be the 'gold standard' (Sackett et al 1997) for research and at the top of a hierarchy of research designs in the development of evidence-based practice guidelines.

FROM PRACTICE TO RESEARCH – STARTING THE RESEARCH PROCESS

Research was defined in Chapter 1 but, however it is defined, research in midwifery aims to directly or indirectly improve midwifery provision to women and their families. Research is *not* an attempt to make every midwife practise in exactly the same way, neither is it an attempt to make every woman experience pregnancy and childbirth identically. It is very unlikely that it would be possible to do either of these things. Research is about identifying the best options for women in a variety of situations, with an understanding of the processes – physical, psychological and social – that may influence that situation. This means that the starting point for midwifery research is usually practice. Regardless of what type of research may eventually be undertaken, there must be an initial idea. This may be triggered by the midwife in practice, reflecting and critically analysing service provision directly or reviewing the literature (Box 2.2).

Box 2.2 Possible questions to trigger research ideas

◆ Why do we do that?
◆ Is A better than B?
◆ What if *x* was done/happened?
◆ How do women feel about *y*?

The same sorts of question are often asked by students trying to develop their knowledge base as they attempt to understand the underlying theories of the events of childbearing that they witness. Women and their families ask the same questions, seeking the rationale behind the various care options. The development of modern drugs, technology and screening processes, both within midwifery and in other health-care disciplines, may suggest new options for women and/or neonates. However, childbearing is a unique human event, which we do not fully understand, and therefore nothing new should be introduced by anyone until it is established that it will at the very least do no harm and hopefully will be of benefit. These are the ethical principles of **nonmaleficence** and **beneficence** (Singleton and McLaren 1995).

Women today want evidence that they are being offered the best care possible, and 'because we've always done it that way' is not an acceptable answer. Women want to make choices for themselves and this is only possible if they have access to the underpinning knowledge and its supporting evidence. This concept of informed choice and control was set out in the report *Changing Childbirth* (Department of Health 1993) and the SNMAC report (Department of Health 1998), which considered the future of midwifery. Therefore, the initial idea for a research study can originate from many sources.

Obtaining the initial idea is not as simple as it sounds. Some practitioners do not fully observe what is actually happening on a daily basis and therefore miss the signs that are shouting: Research me! This could be because of pressure of work or other distractions, including the many workplace and personal stressors. Others see the signs but ignore them, or the ideas are begun but never carried through, much like the fate of the seed in the parable of the sower (Jerusalem Bible 1968, Mark 13: 1–9). Not every midwife has the necessary skills, time or support to undertake research but all should be alert to topics that are in need of evaluation, and to practices that are creeping into daily use without being evaluated. It could be argued that if everything has to be fully researched then imagination would be stifled. In fact, the opposite is true: imagination and creativity are essential to produce the initial research idea. This is not the responsibility of a few research midwives but part of the role of every midwife (UKCC 1998). The research idea may be the result of professional debate and consensus, as in the case of the Delphi survey to establish research priorities in midwifery education (Sleep et al 1995a) or for midwifery practice (Sleep et al 1995b).

As a midwife with a great idea, what do you do with it? The next step is to read about the topic, talk to colleagues, women and friends. Do they all know the answer and are you convinced by their replies? It may be that the information is already available, even though it is new to you. This self-discovery of information is important, as it corresponds to the principle of lifelong learning, and is essential for modern, questioning practitioners (English National Board 1994). In addition, this process of initial enquiry can focus the research topic and help identify the fundamental aspects that need further study.

The next step is huge, and does take courage and self-confidence, characteristics that all midwives should develop. The idea needs to be taken to someone who will either consider it as a potential research topic or help you take it along a research path yourself. Ideally, every maternity unit would have a research and/or development coordinator with whom ideas can be shared and explored. There may even be a research group already conducting research from whom you can seek advice and support. There may be a midwifery forum that welcomes initiatives from staff, which should include research ideas as well as managerial concerns. Alternatively it may be appropriate to approach a manager or supervisor of midwifery, and you should know the route most likely to succeed in your locality. Perseverance may be needed to find the right person or group. Another useful support source may be the local midwifery education establishment. Many schools of midwifery are now within universities, which have a tradition of research; indeed in many universities research is the highest priority. Therefore, midwifery education personnel may be able to either support you in undertaking the research or advise you how the idea can be taken further.

If local support is not available, it may be worth approaching other midwife researchers who have an interest in a similar area. Professional organizations and voluntary groups may also be interested depending on the topic. MIRIAD and MIDIRS are useful resources and could indicate where help might be sought. A well-known midwifery research centre is the National Perinatal Epidemiology Unit; however, they may be fully occupied with current research so it is advisable to start locally.

As part of the idea-formation and support-seeking process it is important to consider whether the topic area would be best investigated by a multi-disciplinary group. This would provide an additional source of support and a pooling of expertise and resources. Collaborative studies are increasingly being encouraged as being an effective way of achieving clinically significant research. The NHS Research and Development (R&D) funds multidisciplinary research studies. The mother and child health initiative launched in 1995 resulted in 51 projects involving a range of professional groups (NHS Executive 1997). Midwifery research is established nationally, with major studies being undertaken in centres such as Bristol, Leeds and Birmingham, to name but a few.

Financial support can be difficult to obtain. Small studies may be self-funded or undertaken as part of the higher degree, with a variety of bodies funding the courses. Funding larger projects can be problematic. There is a high level of competition for funding. Collaborative studies have advantages, in terms of the quality of the submission, due to the collective expertise of the research group, and the increased likelihood of achieving useful data. Again, it is advisable to seek local support first, as NHS trusts increasingly have research and development budgets. Industry and commercial companies may offer support; however, it is important to consider the ethical ramifications of such funding. Many charities offer grants, scholarships and awards of various sizes to researchers and/or specific projects. There are publications available that indicate which bodies offer research awards and their areas of interest. For example, *The Association of Medical Research Charities Handbook* is published annually from 29 Farringdon Road, London, EC1M 3JB. Similar information is available on the Internet. A research-funding database based in Newcastle can be found at www:refund.ncl.ac.uk and a database of biomedical funding agencies can be found at www:wisdom.wellcome.ac.uk/wisdom fundhome.

Finally, there are regional and national research and development bodies that regularly provide research grants, as does the Medical Research Council. The chance of gaining support from these organizations is dependent on two factors:

◆ the quality of the proposal
◆ the perceived significance of the research to practice and health care.

In addition, success may reflect current care and research priorities, so if your research idea reflects a topical health objective it is more likely to receive favourable consideration. The main R&D councils seek research proposals in specific fields and, although these target established research groups rather than individual midwives, it may be useful to find out which areas are current. Midwifery units can help all practitioners to be aware of research issues via a research board where R&D publications as well as topical papers are displayed.

CONCLUSION

Every midwife is the potential trigger for a research project. Questions are generated through personal reflections on practice. This, together with the ability to take the idea further as a potential research project requires the practitioner to have a sound understanding of the research process. When you have the research idea, you then need to consider how the topic could be studied, which research paradigm is most appropriate and which research approach might fulfil the study aims. Exploration of the idea in parallel with consideration of the research process allows for further clarification and, ultimately, high-quality research. The next chapters will consider the main research approaches. These are essential for all midwives, who need to evaluate research papers as part of their practice, but will also help midwives with research ideas to develop them further.

CHAPTER SUMMARY

This chapter has highlighted that:

◆ Research is essential to midwifery

◆ There are different types of knowledge, each of which contributes to midwifery theory and practice

◆ The first step of the research process for the midwife is to gain the idea from practice, followed closely by seeking the support of colleagues locally.

REFERENCES

Benner P 1984 From novice to expert: excellence and power in clinical practice. Addison-Wesley, Menlo Park, CA

Bennett V R, Brown L K 1993 Myles' textbook for midwives, 12th edn. Churchill Livingstone, Edinburgh

Bluff R Ongoing study. Fitting in and staying out of trouble: the influence of midwives on student learning.

Boud D, Keogh R, Walker D 1985 Promoting reflection in learning: a model. In: Boud D, Keogh R, Walker D (ed) Reflection: turning experience into learning. Kogan Page/Nichols, London, ch 1, p 18–40

Bryar R M 1995 Theory for midwifery practice. Macmillan, Basingstoke

Carper B A 1978 Fundamental patterns of knowing in nursing. Advances in Nursing Science 1(1): 13–23

Chinn P L, Kramer M K 1991. Theory and nursing: a systematic approach. Mosby/Year Book, St Louis, MO

Clark E 1987 Sources of nursing knowledge, Research Awareness Module 2. Distance Learning Centre, South Bank Polytechnic, London

Cluett E R, Alexander J, Pickering R 1995 Is measuring the symphysis fundal distance worthwhile? An investigation into the intra-observer and inter-observer variability of abdominal measurement of the distance between the symphysis pubis and the uterine fundus using a paper tape measure. Midwifery 11(4): 174–183

Cormack D F S (ed) 1996 The research process in nursing, 3rd edn. Blackwell Science, Oxford

Department of Health 1993 Changing childbirth. Report of the Expert Maternity Group. HMSO, London

Department of Health 1998 Midwifery: delivering our future. Report by the Standing Nursing and Midwifery Advisory Committee. HMSO, London

Donnison J 1988 Midwives and medical men. A history of the struggle for the control of childbirth. Historical Publication, London

English National Board 1994 Creating lifelong learners: partnerships for care. English National Board for Nursing, Midwifery and Health Visiting, London

Flint C 1986 Sensitive midwifery. Heinemann Nursing, Oxford

Fraser D, Murphy R, Worth-Butler M 1997 An outcome evaluation of the effectiveness of pre-registration midwifery programmes of education. ENB Research Highlights. English National Board for Nursing, Midwifery and Health Visiting No 24, July. ENB, London

Gilbert N 1993 Research, theory and methods. In: Researching social life. Sage Publications, London, ch 2, p 18–31

Hicks C M 1996 Understanding midwifery research. A basic guide to design and analysis. Churchill Livingstone, Edinburgh

Hurley J 1998 Midwives and research-based practice. British Journal of Midwifery 6(5): 294–297

Jackson K 1994 So much for common sense. British Journal of Midwifery 2(3): 131–132

Jerusalem Bible 1968 The Jerusalem Bible (gen ed A Jones). Darton, Longman & Todd, London

Kaplan A 1968 Positivism. In: Sills D L (ed) International encyclopedia of social sciences. Macmillan/Free Press, New York

Kuhn T 1970 The structure of the scientific revolutions, 2nd edn. International Encyclopedia of United States. Chicago University Press, Chicago, IL

Mander R 1992 See how they learn: experience as the basis for practice. Nurse Education Today 12: 11–18

Mulhall A 1994 The experimental approach and randomized controlled trials. In: Hardy M, Mulhall A (ed) Nursing research – theory and practice. Chapman & Hall, London, ch 6, p 103–125

NHS Executive 1997 Mother and child health newsletter. NHS Executive South Thames R & D Directorate

Page L 1997 Evidence based maternity care: science and sensitivity in practice. New Generation Digest 20: 2–3

Parahoo A K 1997 Nursing research. Principles, process and issues. Macmillan, Basingstoke

Paul R W, Heaslip P 1995 Critical thinking and intuitive nursing practice. Journal of Advanced Nursing 22(1): 40–47

Perry A (ed) 1997 Nursing: a knowledge base for practice, 2nd edn. Edward Arnold, London

Phillips T, Bedford H, Robinson J, Schostak J 1994 Researching professional education. Education, dialogue and assessment: creating partnership for improving practice. English National Board for Nursing, Midwifery and Health Visiting, London

Polanyi M 1958 Personal knowledge: towards a post critical philosophy. Routledge & Kegan Paul, London

Polit D F, Hungler B P 1997 Essentials of nursing research. Methods, appraisal and utilization, 4th edn. JB Lippincott, Philadelphia, PA

Reid N 1993 Health care research by degrees. Blackwell Scientific, Oxford

Sackett D L, Richardson W S, Rosenberg W, Haynes R B 1997 Evidence-based medicine. How to practice and teach EBM. Churchill Livingstone, Edinburgh

Schön D A 1983 The reflective practitioner: how professionals think in action. Basic Books/Harper Collins, London

Sidell M 1989 How do we know what we think we know? In: Brechin A, Walmsley J (ed) Making connections: reflecting on the lives and experiences of people with learning difficulties. Hodder & Stoughton in association with the Open University, London, ch 35, p 261–269

Singleton J, McLaren S 1995 Ethical foundations of health care. Responsibilities in decision making. Mosby/Times Mirror International Publishers, London

Sleep J, Bullock I, Grayson K 1995a Establishing priorities for research in education within one college of nursing and midwifery. Nurse Education Today 15(6): 439–445

Sleep J, Renfrew M J, Dunn A, Bowler U, Garcia J 1995b Establishing research priorities for research: report of a Delphi survey. British Journal of Midwifery 3(6): 323–331

Sweet B R 1997 Mayes' midwifery. A textbook for midwives, 12th edn. Baillière Tindall, London

Towler J, Bramall J 1986 Midwives in history and society. Croom Helm, London

UKCC 1998 Midwives' rules and code of practice. United Kingdom Central Council for Nursing, Midwifery and Health Visiting, London

3

Experimental research

Elizabeth Cluett

INTRODUCTION

The experimental research approach is the epitome of the quantitative paradigm. Many health-care advances can be attributed to experimental research, and it is implicit throughout the two volumes of *Effective Care in Pregnancy and Childbirth* (Chalmers et al 1989) that carefully controlled experimental studies provide some of the best evidence for high-quality care for women and their infants. This could be considered a narrow perspective and some, including Sapsford and Abbott (1992) argue that experimental research is limited as it 'artificializes' the real situation. As experimental research, particularly randomized controlled trials, can also have practical difficulties and moral dilemmas (Dawson 1986), it evokes strong, often opposing views. Currently midwifery-related research findings often arise from experimental research and so practitioners need to be able to understand the processes involved, their strengths and limitations. This chapter aims to present a realistic insight into what experimental research can and cannot offer midwifery practice. The experimental research process, the main features of most common designs and midwifery examples are explored.

ORIGINS

It is almost impossible to identify an origin for experimental research. Trial and error could be considered a simple experiment. Science developed increasingly precise ways to conduct, monitor and evaluate the impact of new solutions and these carefully controlled activities, are the foundations of modern experimental research. As Parahoo (1997) points out, everyone uses experimental processes every day. We try out a variety of nonprescription analgesics until we find the most effective one for us. However, the basic experimental design is generally attributed to John Stuart Mill who in 1873, with colleagues, devised a strategy to answer 'what if' questions by recording outcomes to carefully controlled events (Wilson-Barnett 1991). Dawson (1986) and Greenwood (1984) suggest the experimental research processes now used for health-care investigations were derived from botany and agricultural studies. Randomization, the main component in experimental research was first undertaken by a statistician, Fisher, in the 1920s in an agricultural setting (Oakley 1990). The aim was, and still is, to find relationships between actions taken and outcomes seen or experienced. So, although modern experimental research is associated with laboratories, complex equipment and techniques, it is a human way of expanding knowledge and of problem-solving.

THE NATURE OF EXPERIMENTAL RESEARCH – WHAT IT IS AND ITS PURPOSE

Fundamentally an experiment is a test, and experimental research is a quantitative process in which various ideas or concepts are tested. Quantitative research is based on a **positivist** philosophy, in which empirical data is used to explain and increase knowledge about the physical world, of which people are a part. Ideally, precise measurements are obtained, in an objective manner, of each part of the subject, event or process. Parahoo (1997) indicates that quantitative research endeavours to be **deterministic**, meaning that one of the key functions of quantitative research is to determine the presence and magnitude of any relationship between the subjects, events or processes, and ultimately to see if there is evidence of cause and effect (**causal**). Demonstration of such relationships is highly complex and another dimension of quantitative research is therefore its **deductive** nature. This is the process by which a **hypothesis** is proposed, suggesting the relationship between the phenomena, which can then be tested through data collection and analysis until the hypothesis is accepted or rejected. This reductionist approach assumes that each subject, event or process is the sum of its parts. In respect of life, human or otherwise, this is not just a gross over-simplification, but is erroneous when the spiritual, psychological and social dimensions are considered. In addition, it is assumed that the subject, event or process (also known as the **phenomenon**) will not be affected by the process of measuring it or by those undertaking the measurements. Despite its limitations, the use of a reductionist approach does enable the growth of knowledge, by facilitating the division of a large topic into smaller sections that can be explored both practically and conceptually. It is because of these characteristics that the experimental approach has been placed at one end of the research continuum (Chapter 2).

Quantitative research is considered as a hierarchy: experimental research, quasi-experimental research and nonexperimental research. Experimental research is undertaken when a cause-and-effect relationship is being sought. Quasi-experimental research is undertaken when it is not possible to undertake a true experimental study and therefore, while a cause-and-effect relationship may be identified, often a correlational relationship only can be determined. Finally, nonexperimental research can provide descriptions and evidence of correlations between the topics under investigation. As experimental research involves most of the principles and techniques that are used within quantitative research, experimental research will be considered first. This will make comprehension of quasi-experimental designs, which follow in this chapter, easier. Nonexperimental designs are considered in Chapter 4.

COMPONENTS OF EXPERIMENTAL AND QUASI-EXPERIMENTAL RESEARCH

Quantitative research is a logical, stepwise process, where 'process' is not merely a series of tasks but involves exploration of underpinning theories, beliefs and assumptions that influence the selection and use of the knowledge and skills required for undertaking research (Parahoo 1997). The concepts, principles and practicalities of experimental and quasi-experimental designs will be considered in the order in which a midwife researcher would encounter them when undertaking a research project and in the order in which research reports are presented. To some extent, this is artificial, as few individuals or processes function in perfect order. Ideas and/or information inevitably occur out of sequence and as they emerge it may be necessary to go back and reconsider earlier steps. So researchers feel that for every two steps forward there are three steps back.

Views differ on how many stages there are in experimental research, ranging from four to 10 (Burns and Grove 1993, Reid 1993, Parahoo 1997, Polit and Hungler 1997). I will use five steps; however, step 2 has many subdivisions.

Step 1 – the research question

Gaining the research idea from practice was discussed in Chapter 2. This first idea is usually broad and has to be refined into small researchable portions. A good example of this is perineal care; perhaps the initial question was something like: What is the best perineal care and management midwives can offer postnatal women?

A series of research studies have considered many related issues, including warm versus cold bathing (Ramler and Roberts 1986), the impact of exercise (Sleep and Grant 1987), the use of salt in the bath water (Sleep and Grant 1988), topical analgesics (Moore and James 1989) and many more (see Sleep 1990 for a full review on perineal care). This refining is the result of discussion and, very importantly, consideration of the literature on the topic.

The literature review

The literature review prior to experimental research aims to use current evidence to determine the need for, the aims of and the best method of undertaking the proposed research. Burns and Grove (1993) cite 15 purposes of the literature review in quantitative research, but these can be broadly classified into two groups:

◆ literature to gain as much information as possible on the topic
◆ literature to consider how the topic has been researched previously.

The topic information will include consideration of what is already known, the quality of evidence on which that knowledge is based, and any omissions. This identifies if there is a need for further information and hence a research study.

The literature helps decide what outcomes are measured, and how, to ensure that they are appropriate and that any potentially negative as well as positive effects are identified. Johnson (1997) suggests that studies should be designed to facilitate the collection of long-term outcomes as well as short-term ones, particularly in relation to infant wellbeing. A short-term outcome is a characteristic that is measurable at the time of the research, such as length of labour or amount of analgesia used for perineal postpartum pain. Long-term outcomes would be the sequelae measured 6 months, a year or even many years later, such as dyspareunia 1 year postpartum for a perineal management study.

Secondly, information is gleaned from the literature as to which aspects of the designs were successful or unsuccessful, the objective being to improve future research designs. To achieve these aims a wide variety of literature should be considered, including primary sources. These are articles, papers, reports that are original documents, such as research studies and their findings, retrospective studies, case studies and audit information. Even within these primary sources there is a hierarchy, with the greatest credence being given to research findings. Secondary sources include literature reviews, commentaries and editorials on the topic or on the primary sources. These can be valuable in assisting with critiquing the primary sources, considering opposing perspectives and thus coming to conclusions about the way forward. Letters in journals can be either primary or secondary sources, but often indicate what issues are of concern within the profession and thus may highlight important points to consider.

Accessing the literature is a time-consuming and often frustrating process. Ayres (1995) provides an overview of literature sources. Sources would include direct access to journals via local and national libraries, the use of databases such as the Cochrane Pregnancy and Childbirth Database, CINAHL, MIRIAD and Medline. Some databases do not maintain a full index of all published studies; for example, Medline currently indexes approximately 40% of literature. Hawkins (1997) provides an introduction to using databases. Bibliographic services such as MIDIRS, the Royal College of Midwives' Current Awareness service, offer prepared bibliographies and personal searches. Each article's reference list can be useful to focus on specific points and gain other sources. Further trawls refine the precise research question and method. It is vital that all the literature, including obscure journals, is critiqued, which can be time-consuming. Time and effort invested increase the chances of success. If you have access to the Worldwide Web, then under-taking a search on Medline, the premier medical index (Toth 1997), is free and has been designed to be user-friendly.

It is important to review as much literature as possible to avoid obtaining a biased perspective. However, it should be noted that there is a tendency for studies with positive results to be published while others are not. This can bias the availability of literature on a topic.

Research variables and hypothesis formation

The 'what' and 'outcomes' to be studied, identified from the literature, are the research variables, where variables are characteristics or facets of the research topic between which a relationship is suspected. If there was no suggestion of a relationship between these characteristics/facets, there would be no need for the research. There are two types of variable: **independent** and **dependent** variables (Box 3.1).

Box 3.1 Examples of independent and dependent variables

Does one-to-one midwifery care reduce the length of labour?

◆ One-to-one midwifery care is the independent variable

◆ Length of labour is the dependent variable

Do neonates cry more if delivered into bright light?

◆ The bright light is the independent variable

◆ The amount of crying is the dependent variable.

Note that in the second question the variables are in the opposite order, so it is important to identify which characteristic is the cause and which the outcome.

To prevent confusion, remember that experimental research is about cause and effect. So the independent variable is the cause and is what is being tested by the study. The dependent variable is the effect, i.e. the outcome that will be measured.

Extraneous or **confounding** variables refer to any eventuality that could affect the research outcome accidentally. They are not in the research question but may be identified within any discussion of the research design, highlighting whether they were predicted or came to light during the research process. For example, these might be environmental factors, the time of day or day of the week, people or equipment.

Where variables have the potential to be interpreted differently by practitioners, working definitions must be given, sometimes known as research definitions, or research terms. This means that it does not matter if the day of delivery is called day 0 or day 1, so long as it is clearly defined for the study. This allows midwives practising in areas where the alternative definition is used to interpret the results as they would be applied to their situation.

Research can be posed as a question:

One-to-one midwifery care may affect the length of labour.

Does one-to-one midwifery care reduce the length of labour?

In experimental research it is normal practice to word the question as a **hypothesis**, making it easier to test than a question. A hypothesis is a statement of the proposed relationship between the given variables. There are several ways the hypothesis can be expressed: the first is as a simple one-directional hypothesis, which states the relationship and its direction. Parahoo (1997) states that this type of research hypothesis indicates what the results will show. Thus the question above would become:

One-to-one midwifery care reduces the length of labour.

Predicting the results in this way may not be possible or could result in other effects being missed or cause researcher bias. It is preferable to have a nondirectional or neutral hypothesis, which would be:

One-to-one midwifery care may affect the length of labour.

This can be developed one step further to a **null hypothesis**. This is the preferred option for experimental research, for statistical reasons. It is almost impossible to prove anything for certain. Consider birthweight: it could be proposed that the biggest baby to deliver vaginally was 5.2 kg. To prove this, every baby in the world would need to be weighed, and there is always the baby due tomorrow. However the hypothesis would be relatively easy to disprove by finding a baby weighing 5.3 kg, clearly a much more realistic task. Thus null or negative statements, which can be disproved, are considered more appropriate for experimental research. The null hypothesis suggests there is *no* relationship between variables. So the original question becomes:

One-to-one midwifery care makes no difference to the length of labour.

The final type of hypothesis that may be used is the complex hypothesis, which is where more than one outcome is being considered. For example:

One-to-one midwifery care makes no difference to the length of labour or maternal satisfaction with labour.

So the initial research idea is now a precise research hypothesis, ready for testing through an experimental design. The next step is planning that design, but first try converting the following research questions into null hypotheses and identify the independent and dependent variables (Box 3.2).

> **Box 3.2** Hypothesis formation
>
> **Try converting these research questions into null hypotheses to check your understanding**
> ◆ Does aromatherapy during labour decrease pain experience and the use of pethidine?
> ◆ Can tea bags reduce nipple pain in breastfeeding women?
> ◆ Would attending five study days per year increase midwives' knowledge and skill?
> The answers can be found at the end of the chapter.

Step 2 – Planning the study design

The literature review will inform the decisions as to which is the most appropriate design for the study. To refine the study, experts in the relevant design and advisors such as medical statisticians and epidemiologists can be consulted. These personnel may not have midwifery knowledge but can usually guide the design process to ensure that findings obtained are reliable and valid. The main designs will now be considered in turn.

Three key concepts in experimental research

The true experiment has three characteristics: manipulation, control and randomization (Pocock 1983). These are all present in the randomized controlled trial (RCT).

Manipulation is the purposeful introduction of some form of intervention. This might be a treatment, such as in the ORACLE study, where the value of antibiotics in the management of idiopathic preterm labour is being investigated (ORACLE Clinical Coordinating Centre 1996). It could equally be a new information leaflet, such as a postnatal exercise sheet, or a new care environment, such as a natural birth room. Throughout this chapter the term 'intervention group' will be used to identify the group that is receiving the new management/care/treatment. Other authors may use the term treatment or study group.

Control can be seen as a negative concept, particularly in midwifery, where the emphasis is on enabling women to be in control of their childbirth experiences. Keeble (1995) explores the issues of control in relation to the researcher, the participant and the research process. She concludes that properly conducted experimental research does not remove participants' control of events and in the long term may contribute additional knowledge that may enable others to have greater control (Keeble 1995). Control refers to two separate issues within the research process. Firstly, it involves the controlling of various facets of the research, such as the environment in which it is conducted, criteria for participants and how the data is obtained and analysed, all of which should be specified in the research protocol (Polit and Hungler 1997). Secondly, the **control group** is the comparison group of participants, who are drawn from the same population as the intervention group and are thus the same in every way except that they do not receive the intervention. Thus, any difference found between the groups must be attributable to the intervention. Traditionally, the control group was equated with a no-treatment group or a group receiving a placebo. Collier (1995) and Ernst and Resch (1995) discuss ethical and practical implications of 'no treatment' versus 'placebo' groups. As it would be unethical to deprive women and/or infants of any known beneficial intervention, the control group usually refers to the group receiving the best current management or treatment, while the intervention group receives the new or trial intervention.

Randomization is the allocation of subjects to either the intervention or control group by chance. The aim is to ensure that the groups are comparable in all characteristics other than the management options under study. Thus the distribution of characteristics such as age, ethnic origin, educational attainment should be equal across all groups. There are several methods of randomizing individuals to study groups, described extensively by Pocock (1983); the simplest is to flip a coin. More appropriate and convenient are statistical texts, which give tables of randomized numbers that can be used, or recent practice is to use computer-generated random numbers. This facilitates a prestudy randomization plan, which removes any opportunity for bias through the influence of the researchers or participants. Once the computer has generated the random allocation of subjects, the information is transferred to sealed opaque envelopes by someone not involved in the data collection, so the randomization cannot be broken prior to subject recruitment. For multicentre studies a telephone system may be used whereby, at the point of recruitment, the local practitioner rings the administration centre and is given the randomized allocation.

There is a possibility that random allocation could result in groups of unequal numbers. This is likely to be insignificant in studies involving large numbers but may be of concern in smaller studies. **Block randomization** ensures that the distribution of participants to each arm of the trial is equal after a specified number of individuals have been recruited, yet the allocation remains random and cannot be predicted by the researchers (Pocock 1983). For example, if the study is to have only 30 participants, 15 in the intervention group and 15 in the control group, randomization in blocks of 10 would mean that, after every 10 individuals had been recruited, 5 would be in the intervention group and 5 in the control group.

The concept of **blinding**, while not one of the defining characteristics of experimental research, is one that is recommended to reduce bias (Pocock 1983). There are two levels of blinding. Double blinding, where neither participants nor researcher(s) know which arm of the trial or group allocation the participant is in, is the option adopted most often in drug trials, where it is feasible to produce identical treatment packages for all participants regardless of which arm of the study the individual is allocated to. Single blinding describes the situation where the participant does not know whether she is in the intervention or the control group, but those collecting the data and conducting the study do.

The advantage of blinding is the avoidance of inadvertent preferential treatment for one group over another. Participants can all believe they have received the treatment option perceived to be best; thus psychological influences, including motivational factors, should be equalized across all groups. The importance of psychological influences on research has been known since the identification of the Hawthorne effect (Roethlisberger and Dickson 1939). Hawthorne was the name of an electrical company in which productivity increased regardless of what change was instigated; thus the change was due to the research process and not to the actual changes. In a double-blind study where there are apparently identical intervention packages the Hawthorne effect can be considered as equal across groups; any difference in outcome measures must therefore be due to the intervention. In many studies, treatments cannot be blinded. Within midwifery it may be argued that most studies cannot be double-blinded and the implication of this must be explored in the research findings.

In studies where there is double blinding, it may become essential to break the blinding to identify whether a particular individual is receiving the treatment or placebo – for instance, in drug trials, if the participant is admitted to hospital and there is a possibility that his/her condition is related to the study. So there must always be provision for a central office or person, not directly involved with the data collection, to be able to identify which arm of the study the individual is in. In less severe circumstances, for example where the study treatment could impact on a subsequent treatment, then the individual is withdrawn from the study and care is provided appropriate to his/her needs. For example, in the ORACLE study, any woman who was considered to need antibiotics for clinical reasons would be withdrawn and prescribed the appropriate antibiotics. Thus breaking the code would not be necessary.

The sample: selection, inclusion criteria and size

Ideally all women who met the study criteria would be recruited into the study; thus the sample would be a **total population**. The best-known example of a total population study is the decennial census of the population, involving questionnaires to every household in the country, carried out by the Office of Population Census and Surveys (OPCS). OPCS surveys are nonexperimental research designs. To achieve total population samples in experimental research requires very large studies and this is often not possible. One major difficulty is accessing the population. Imagine, for example, a study considering the benefits of a new format for parentcraft sessions compared to the traditional classes for primigravid women. A total population would be all primigravid women; however, many women decide not to attend any classes, some work and are unable to attend at the appropriate times, while others may have obstetric complications that result in preterm delivery. Thus from the total population there is a subgroup of women suitable for inclusion to the study. This subgroup can be called the **study population** or the target population. The study population is defined for each research project by the **inclusion criteria**. These are unique to each research project. Some researchers give **exclusion criteria** – in other words, who from the whole population is not suitable or is protected, such as potentially vulnerable groups like under-16-year-olds. Research that focuses on vulnerable groups must take their needs into account and justification of their inclusion becomes a key ethical consideration (Kennell et al 1991). The importance of identifying the correct inclusion criteria cannot be overemphasized. If the study population includes inappropriate participants, the validity of the study may be questioned. For example the Bristol Third Stage Trial (Prendiville et al 1988) considered a care option for low-risk women, physiological management of the third stage of labour, but included women at increased risk of post-partum haemorrhage in a study where the incidence of haemorrhage was a key outcome measure. Thus the applicability of the research findings to low-risk women is in question.

Even where the study population has been defined it may not be possible to involve all potential participants because of their large number and/or the practicalities of accessing and undertaking experimental research on that size of population. In addition it may be possible to answer the research question and obtain significant results without involving an entire study population. It is not ethical to involve more participants than is necessary to achieve the aims of the study. A second benefit of using a smaller sample is the reduction in cost.

Where a population sample is not possible/necessary, random selection or **probability sampling** is recommended for all quantitative research designs. This means that a subset of the defined population is selected, so that every member has a known chance of being recruited. This ensures that the sample is representative of the total population, which is essential if the results are to be generalizable to the wider population and considered reliable and valid (Meinert and Tonascia 1986). Ideally, bias due to constraints such as specific day of the week or time of day, or preference for approachable individuals, should not be possible. Thus the two main aims of any sampling method are to:

◆ maximize the representativeness of the sample to the study population
◆ minimize the potential for any bias.

The four recognized probability sampling methods are:

◆ simple randomization
◆ stratified random sampling
◆ systematic sampling
◆ convenience sampling.

Simple randomization is where each member of the study population has an equal chance of being recruited to the study. This is achieved using random numbers, either from a table or generated by a computer. For example, imagine a study considering the value of loaning a TENS machine to women at 37 weeks gestation. First, the number of women required to obtain useful results would be calculated. Let's use 20 for this example. Then the number of women of 37 weeks gestation attending the maternity unit during the research period would be calculated, say 100 for this example. The table or computer then generates a list of random numbers, up to 20, from a 100 block, as indicated by the shaded boxes in Figure 3.1.

Every women has the same chance of being selected, a 1 in 5 chance, but

1	2	3	4	5	6	7	8	9	10
11	12	13	14	15	16	17	18	19	20
21	22	23	24	25	26	27	28	29	30
31	32	33	34	35	36	37	38	39	40
41	42	43	44	45	46	47	48	49	50
51	52	53	54	55	56	57	58	59	60
61	62	63	64	65	66	67	68	69	70
71	72	73	74	75	76	77	78	79	80
81	82	83	84	85	86	87	88	89	90
91	92	93	94	95	96	97	98	99	100

Figure 3.1 A random number table

only the highlighted women will be asked to participate in the study. This is very similar to how random allocation to trial study groups is achieved. This method of sampling assumes that every woman has the same characteristics. Thus in the example used here, which could include primigravid and multigravid participants, it is possible that, by chance there is an unequal number of primigravidae compared to multigravidae. This can be overcome by using stratified random sampling.

Stratified sampling enables researchers to achieve samples that have the same proportion of stated characteristics as are present in the whole population. This is sometimes called proportional sampling. Thus in the example above, if 60% of the women are multigravid and 40% primigravid, the sample for the study would mirror the 60/40 split. This is achieved by effectively having two sets of random numbers, one for primigravidae and one for multigravidae, with 12 (60%) and 8 (40%) women being selected for each group respectively. This can be repeated for as many characteristics as is considered appropriate, but it should reflect characteristics that are likely to have an impact on the outcomes being measured. So in a study about TENS affecting pain, clinical experience would suggest that parity would affect this outcome, whereas height or eye colour would not. Thus it is important that decisions related to sampling methods are based on clinical knowledge. A knowledge of the research process alone is not sufficient.

Systematic sampling is where every nth person is approached to achieve the required sample size as a percentage of the total. For example if the study requires 50% of the population then every second woman would be approached. This sampling method is very simple to organize and execute but can lead to potential bias; for example, every 10th women might be delivered during the night, or at weekends. This type of bias is known as systematic bias and this form of sampling is therefore best avoided.

Convenience sampling is the use of a sample that is readily available or easy to access. It is often used where recruitment only occurs when specific researchers are available. In large studies this is not a problem, as there should be researchers available at all times. In small studies, where the number of personnel able to recruit is restricted, this sampling method can lead to systematic bias, particularly if the recruiting midwife works set hours. Research has to be conducted within the real-life situation, and therefore there are occasions when convenience sampling is the only option available. The limitations should be noted by both researchers and those reading subsequent reports, when considering any research findings.

Sample size

The aim of any experimental research is to achieve results that can be generalized from the sample to the whole target population. This can only be done if the sample is large enough to ensure that it is representative of the population and achieve significance in the statistical analysis. The calculation of sample size, called **power calculations**, should be undertaken by a statistician. In general, the less common the outcome measured the greater the sample size needed to achieve significance. For example, fetal death is relatively rare; therefore to test the effect of a new care option on the incidence of fetal death many thousands of participants would be needed. Alternatively, perineal trauma is fairly common, so a study to see if a new care option affected the incidence of perineal trauma would require a smaller sample.

Outcome measures that are discrete events generally require larger sample sizes than continuous data. For example, to show if waterbirth reduces the use of epidural anaesthesia would require a greater number of women in the sample than a study that asked women to indicate their pain level on a 0–10 score and was looking for a reduction in that score. The magnitude of the difference in the expected outcome measure between the trial group and control group also affects the sample size. For example, if providing one-to-one care is expected to result in a 20% reduction in epidural anaesthesia, a small sample would be able to detect this large difference. However, it is rare that such large differences would be expected, so where there is only a relatively small difference in the outcome measure between groups, say a 5% difference, a much larger sample size is needed.

The researchers and the research environment

It is important that personnel designing the study and undertaking the data collection process are suitably qualified and prepared. This includes initial and ongoing training and support.

The research environment is usually the clinical area, and ensuring that clinical care is protected is paramount. The practicalities of conducting studies within the clinical environment mean that experienced practitioners should always be involved in the planning stages and piloting should always be done to identify any areas of concern.

The randomized controlled trial (RCT)

A meticulously designed and executed RCT is the gold standard of quantitative research (Gallo et al 1995). It aims to demonstrate the presence or absence and magnitude of any causal relationship between the factor(s) under investigation. With precise statistical analysis an indication of the reliability and the inferred generalizability can be attributed to the study results. The strengths, considered by Wilson-Barnett (1991), are achieved by controlling or equalizing all extraneous variables across groups (a control group and one or more intervention groups), using the three key concepts described earlier. It could be argued that RCTs are the only effective way to ensure that current obstetric and midwifery practice is evidence-based. The development of the Cochrane Databases in obstetrics, and now in other medical domains, is based on this assumption. The Department of Health (1992) has acknowledged the importance of RCTs in the evaluation of health technologies by recommending that trials be conducted on all new or existing technologies where their effects have not yet been established. Baum (1993) goes further, suggesting that the need for health care based on RCTs is so great that the entire population should be encouraged to demand that their care has been fully researched in this manner. To support this, he advocates that everyone should agree to participate in such trials (Baum 1993). This proactive philosophy appears similar to that of organ donation cards, in that individuals agree in principle to RCTs prior to the onset of any condition that may be the subject of a trial. Enforcing that initial agreement at the time of possible recruitment is a different ethical dilemma. However, such suggestions emphasize the value attributed to the RCT by its proponents.

In contrast, it could be argued that the RCT gives a false image of objectivity and that the controlling and reductionist approach of any RCT fails to appreciate the unique nature of the person. A more humanistic philosophy might suggest that, because human nature is so complex, any supposed outcome from an RCT that is a causal relationship is at best tentative and possibly erroneous, being as much the result of interactions, real or perceived, between the study process and participants as of the treatments under consideration.

There are a variety of designs within the overall classification of RCTs. The variations may influence the type and quality of the information gained. Schwartz and Lellouch (1967) identified two broad approaches to RCTs, explanatory and pragmatic. The former aims primarily to enhance knowledge and the latter to inform the decision-making processes related to medical treatment. The pragmatic approach attempts to evaluate a series of management options for a particular group, in order to determine the best care options in a given set of circumstances. Midwives are most likely to be involved in studies using the pragmatic approach, as they are carried out in the clinical environment. The design recognizes that treatments and people are complex, that study participants are a specific group identified prior to the study and that withdrawals from the study are anticipated, and the analysis aims to ensure that errors could not result in the treatments/managements being worse than stated (Schwartz and Lellouch 1967). The explanatory approach is analogous to the laboratory experiment where only those who actually receive the stipulated intervention are included in the analysis, which aims to identify any change in outcomes regardless of direction or magnitude.

The traditional RCT design

The traditional design for an RCT can be represented by Fig. 3.2. This diagram has been based on the trial designs detailed in Pocock (1983), Meinert and Tonascia (1986) and Parmar (1992).

There are difficulties with obtaining informed consent before randomization, which has led to a variety of designs that randomize before consent – a randomized consent design (Zelen 1979), in which only those receiving the intervention know of the study, or a two-sided consent model, where participants are randomized and then consent is sought for the option to which they have been allocated (Zelen 1990, Parmar 1992). In self-allocation designs, those willing to be randomized are allocated but participants not willing to be randomly allocated are self-allocated (Brewin and Bradley 1989, Silverman 1994). Each of these designs has significant advantages and disadvantages in terms of ethics, research credibility and practicalities, which are considered by the authors cited. Oakley (1990) discusses their compatibility with feminist principles. There is debate as to the value of these designs within experimental research, which is beyond the scope of this text but does highlight the fact that experimental research design is not static but open for review and development to meet the changing needs of society.

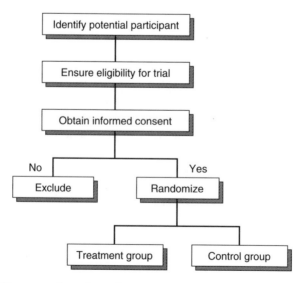

Figure 3.2 Diagram to show the traditional randomized controlled trial design

Post-test-only design

This is a simple yet good design. Participants are selected using a probability sampling method, then randomly allocated to the intervention and control groups. The outcomes are measured and compared across groups. This design measures outcomes that are single events, such as mode of delivery, use of epidural anaesthesia or admission to the neonatal unit. However, there is no measure of change. So if pain levels in women using TENS or a mock unit were being considered, a lower score in the TENS group might just reflect the fact that this group of women had a lower pain experience, not that TENS machines were reducing pain levels.

Pre- and post-test designs

The research process is the same as the group above, except that the outcome variables under investigation are measured before the intervention as well as after it. Thus, returning to the TENS example, pain scores would be recorded prior to the use of the TENS/mock machines as well as after it. Then the degree of change can be compared and directly attributed to the intervention. This design can be problematic if the measurement process involves a questionnaire or testing process where participants may learn from the process of the questionnaire/test. Any perceived change might be due to the assessment process rather than the actual intervention.

Solomon Four design

This design aims to overcome the difficulties with both the preceding designs by having elements of both. It is a randomized controlled trial, with appropriate probability sampling; however random allocation is to four groups. This can be described by Table 3.1.

Table 3.1 The Solomon Four design of RCT	
Allocation type	**Outcomes measured**
Control group	After study period only
Control group	Before and after study period
Intervention group	After intervention only
Intervention group	Before and after intervention

Now it is possible to analyse both the impact of the intervention and the impact of the measurement processes involved in the study. This is a more complex design. The main disadvantages include the greater number of participants required and the fact that, if there are significant differences in the numbers in each arm of the study, the results could be biased. It is more difficult to organize, requiring more administration, equipment and personnel, and is therefore more expensive.

Factorial designs

Factorial design enables the comparison of more than one independent variable and consideration of the interaction of the variables. In addition, significant results can be achieved with a smaller sample size than if each facet was considered individually (Pocock 1983). As with all RCTs, there should be probability sampling and random allocation to the intervention/control groups. A good example of a factorial design in midwifery is the study conducted by Alexander (1996) into breastfeeding rates in women with inverted or non-protractile nipples. This can be described by Table 3.2, which is a 2 by 2 table.

Table 3.2 Study groups in the factorial design used by Alexander (1996)

● Exercise and breast shells	● Exercises only
● Breast shells only	● No intervention

Analysis would be possible for the following factors:

◆ the effect of exercises compared to no intervention on breastfeeding rates
◆ the effect of breast shells compared to no invention on breastfeeding rates
◆ the effect of exercises and shells compared to no intervention on breastfeeding rates
◆ the effect of exercises compared to breast shells on breastfeeding rates
◆ the effect of exercises and shells compared to exercises alone on breastfeeding rates
◆ the effect of exercises and shells compared to shells alone on breastfeeding rates.

As the list demonstrates there is the potential for many factors to be considered in isolation and in various combinations. It is possible to have 2 by 3 or 3 by 3 factorial designs, with the complexity of the analysis increasing with each increase in factor size. Polit and Hungler (1997) suggest that designs greater than 4 by 4 are unlikely because of the difficulties with analysis and the practical difficulties of recruiting adequate numbers to each factor cell.

Although the above four experimental designs are the ones most commonly used, they are not exclusive. New designs are always being considered in response to new problems. The aims remain the same, to ensure representativeness, reduce bias through random selection and allocation, and achieve careful control of as many facets as possible.

Matched-pair designs

Parahoo (1997) and Reid (1993) consider matched pairs along with experimental research designs. The study population is matched into pairs for key characteristics such as age, parity, education achievements or whatever extraneous variables the researchers wish to control for. Then one of the pair is allocated to the intervention group and the other to the control group, the decision being made at random, again using random tables or a computer. If either one of the pair withdraws from the study then the complete pair is withdrawn. Achieving a good match is very rare as it is difficult to accurately match participants for all the characteristics that may influence the study. It could be argued that this design is another form of sample selection and thus a true experiment. However an alternative view is that the randomization process has been tampered with and that therefore this is not a true experiment. I have therefore put this design between true experiments and quasi-experiments in recognition of the slightly different allocation process.

Quasi-experimental designs

A quasi-experimental design could be described as a design that has only some of the elements of the true experiment. An early understanding of the quasi-experimental design suggested that such designs consisted of manipulation(s) and a controlled process but no randomization (Cook and Campbell 1979), for either ethical or practical reasons. If there was no manipulation (intervention) it would not be an experiment, and such designs are considered separately in Chapter 4. Thus the definition of a quasi-experimental design would be an experiment without random allocation to the study groups. As a result, quasi-designs are considered to be weaker than true experiments. It is difficult to ascertain a cause-and-effect relationship between variables in a quasi-experimental design, as any outcomes may be due to the natural groupings and not to the intervention. Thus their influence on practice must be less.

Nonequivalent groups

A commonly used quasi-experimental design is where there is a comparison group, but it cannot be called a control group because it may not have been selected from the study population, or allocation to the groups may not have been random. This is most like to occur where management options are the focus of the research. For example a study might consider the impact of breastfeeding rates of rooming breastfeeding mothers separately from those artificially feeding their infants. As it may not be possible to have both scenarios in one unit or ward, the woman's allocation might depend on where she lives or who her consultant is. There may be factors that are different for each unit, such as the level of education attainment characteristic of the respective catchment areas or staffing levels in the units, both of which could affect breastfeeding rates.

Practical considerations may also result in natural groups. For example, in their study of the use of enemas in labour, Romney and Gordon (1981) made use of consultant protocols that resulted in women under the care of one obstetrician receiving enemas while those under the care of another did not. Because of these limitations, Drayton and Rees (1989) re-examined the use of enemas in labour with a randomized controlled trial.

Rees (1997) suggests that within midwifery one reason nonequivalent groups may be used is because it is unacceptable to deny women choice related to their care. However it is just as unacceptable to offer choices that have not been researched.

Time series designs

A time series study is one where participants are retested on a number of occasions over a set period of time. If possible, it is advisable to obtain several preintervention tests to establish if the feature under consideration is stable over time. The intervention is then implemented and the postintervention tests are undertaken. Time series designs may or may not have comparison groups. They share the same limitation as other quasi-experimental designs in that they lack randomization; however, an additional disadvantage is that time itself becomes a variable. The longer the study period the more difficult it is to differentiate between the effects of time and those of the intervention.

Natural experiments

These could be considered a form of quasi-experimental design. Two groups are identified, of which one experiences a naturally occurring event and is compared to the other group, which does not have the 'event'. It could be the same group over time, comparing variables before and after the 'event'.

Ex post facto designs

These designs explore what might have influenced outcomes after the events. This type of study has much in common with audit and nonexperimental research. It is, however, a search for new information and can be classified as a partial experiment because an element of intervention is identified and comparisons are made between individuals who received the intervention and those who did not. There is no random allocation to the groups, and the criteria for the groups are identified after the event, so this is a **retrospective** study. The greatest danger is that, as the groups were not selected or allocated in the study, there may be characteristics that account for any differences found. Therefore it is not possible to make firm conclusions about any cause-and-effect relationship from ex post facto designs.

One-group-only designs

In this type of design there is no control group. The reasons for this are usually ethical or practical. One-group designs may be used as a preliminary study prior to a full experimental research project, although there should be clear justification why it is not possible to move directly to an RCT. Within this design there can be post-testing only, or pre- and post-testing. In addition, there could be **crossover designs**. This is where individuals act as their own control. There is a period of intervention and a period of no intervention and the differences are compared. The disadvantage of this design is that there has been no controlling for the research process effects, the Hawthorne effect, and thus any change could be due to the interest of the researchers and not to the intervention. In addition, any change may be due to the natural progression of time, and there is no way of knowing if the intervention/non-intervention periods have influenced each other.

Experimental case studies

There are a few conditions that are so rare that it is impossible to accrue enough participants for a traditional research study. There are also occasions where the extreme nature of a condition means that it may be appropriate to try a new and potentially life-saving intervention that has not been the subject of a true experimental study. In both these cases an experiment is being conducted, and it is research, as measurements pre- and postintervention are recorded. Yet such research cannot meet the criteria for experimental research designs. The main issue is ethical. Participants must be aware of the nature of the intervention and the limited available knowledge about its effects. Any findings have great potential for bias, but such case studies are still worthy of reporting and documenting. They may lead to future developments, which can be the subject of full-scale trials, or, over a period of time, may contribute to the care and management of individuals with rare conditions.

Measurement tools

In experimental research there is always some form of measurement. The tools can vary from technological equipment to measure biophysical data, through data forms to record measurable outcomes such as length of labour, to self-completed questionnaires to record and measure psychosocial data. There is no limit to what may be the research tool, but the following should be considered.

♦ Who designed the tool?
♦ Has it has been used before in other studies?
♦ Does it measure what is required/what it is supposed to measure, i.e. is it valid?
♦ Is it easily used and available for use in the study?
♦ Is it accurate/consistent in use, i.e. is it reliable?

In addition intra- and inter-rater variability needs to be considered. **Intrarater variability** is the degree to which one person obtains the same results when taking the same measurement repeatedly. **Inter-rater variability** is the amount of agreement achieved when different people undertake the measurement. Cluett et al (1995) evaluated intra- and inter-variability when measuring the distance between the symphysis pubis and the uterine fundus postnatally. They found that the level of variability was so great that there could no reliability or validity in the measurement as an indicator of uterine involution. Intra- and inter-rater variability can be reduced through tight procedural guidelines for the undertaking of measurements and by careful preparation of anyone involved in the collection of data. The concepts of reliability and validity are considered in more detail in Chapter 4.

The data is always recorded on a form. When designing this form it is useful to consider whether coding the data is appropriate; usually measurements that relate to categories or names of events are coded, such as male/female, normal delivery/operative delivery. Data that is a precise value is not coded, such as length of labour or volume of blood lost. Coding is the process by which a numerical value is allocated to a specific response. The code can then be entered into the statistical analysis package being used. Coding in advance of data collection can save considerable time later. However, great care is necessary to ensure that all possible responses are coded, as omissions complicate analysis.

The transition from planning to implementation

Consideration of any ethical implications must be ongoing throughout the study, in particular whether harm might be caused directly or indirectly. Indirect harm may be due to increasing participant stress by the research process or raising expectations of the possibility of new treatments/care options, which are then not met. Alternatively, participants' belief in the current care and/or carers could be undermined by implying that the traditional management is not appropriate or that professionals do not know what care is best. It is a requirement that all experimental or quasi-experimental research, which by definition involves an intervention, needs to be considered by a local ethics committee. The role of the ethics committee is to act as gate-keepers to protect the wellbeing of all research participants (Box 3.3). This is in line with the Declaration of Helsinki (World Medical Association 1989).

Box 3.3 The main aims of an Ethics Committee

Guidelines from the Department of Health (1991)

◆ Maintain ethical standards

◆ Protect research subjects from harm

◆ Preserve the rights of the research subjects

◆ Protect researchers from unjustified criticism

◆ Not hinder research without good cause

The guidelines suggest a fine balance, which is best achieved through meticulously designed studies. There are different local ethics committees throughout the country; however, the main information that they require prior to approval of a study is similar. Usually, a detailed form is supplied, requesting information such as that identified in Box 3.4.

Box 3.4 Information likely to be requested by a local Ethics Committee

◆ Title

◆ Research aims/hypothesis

◆ Background/literature review, including any feasibility studies

◆ Subjects, including sample size, inclusion/exclusion criteria

◆ Details on any intervention, particularly of any drugs or medical technologies involved

◆ Details on data collection and analysis

◆ Safety issues, including any perceived risks or ethical issues

◆ Confidentiality

◆ Expertise of researchers

◆ Potential benefits/resourcing effects on service provision

Ethics committees developed alongside medical research, which adopted a quantitative paradigm. The forms reflect this and therefore qualitative researchers may experience some difficulty in completing them. There is usually a nursing/midwifery advisor for each committee, who can be consulted.

Only after ethical approval is obtained can the research move on to the next step, which is conducting the study.

The planning phase involves many decisions. Some have clinical foundations, others are based on research principles; both have the potential to alter the research process and hence any findings. By being aware of this influence a potential weakness can become a strength. Keeble (1995, p. 93) incorporates the many decisions made during experimental research within a flow chart, which could act as a useful checklist not only for those undertaking this type of research but also for those wishing to enhance their knowledge of this research process. At the end of this phase there should be a clear research protocol, which sets out exactly how the research is to be conducted. It must articulate every study detail so that other researchers could duplicate the study.

Step 3 – The empirical phase

Having spent a considerable time designing the research, the next step is to start the empirical phase, i.e. to commence the data collection. Data collection can be divided into:

◆ the pilot study
◆ the main study.

A **pilot study** is a small-scale version of the full trial, using a limited number of participants from the study population. When a total population is being targeted for the main study, using individuals from the same group may contaminate the field. So an alternative but closely matched pilot sample should be selected. The pilot should be conducted with as much care and attention to detail as the main study, because the quality of the pilot will be reflected in the quality of the main study. Pilot information may identify possible outcomes and therefore contribute to the detailed planning of the analysis processes, which are the next stage. From detailed analysis of the pilot study fine adjustments can be made to the main study (Box 3.5). If substantial changes result from the pilot, redesigning the main study may be required, which will involve reconsideration of all the important points, including gaining ethics committee approval and conducting a second pilot study.

Finally, the main study can be commenced. This means meticulously following the research protocol and documenting everything that happens during the study, including successes and errors as these can affect the validity of the findings. During long studies, it is important to keep the team motivated, with updates on recruitment or interesting events. New personnel must receive the same degree of preparation as initial workers to ensure reliability in the data collection methods. During this stage the key skills required of the researchers are leadership and organizational ones.

> **Box 3.5** Aims of a pilot study
>
> ◆ Test the research process in the practice setting
> ◆ Test any measurement instruments (these may have been tested separately before the pilot as well)
> ◆ Assess the feasibility of the research process, including its acceptability to the study population
> ◆ Identify any impact on the clinical environment
> ◆ Finalize costings, including time involved, administration and organizational issues

Stopping a study

Very occasionally an experimental study has to be stopped prior to its completion, for ethical reasons. This is most likely to happen if there is evidence that the intervention has detrimental side-effects and it is therefore unethical to expose more individuals. If the results are overwhelmingly beneficial, then not to offer the intervention to all women would also be unethical. In small and/or local studies such information may become evident during the data collection process and it may become impossible to recruit to the study, as participants and/or practitioners may refuse to accept the less favourable option. In large studies, particularly multicentre studies, it is important that there is a planned intermediate analysis point, which will consider whether it is safe and ethical to continue. Such interim findings are undertaken by experts outside the study, and are not usually published if the study continues. The aim is to safeguard the wellbeing of future participants. A safety protocol, which identifies data to be collected to monitor safety, should be part of the main research protocol. This must include specifying who is responsible for terminating a study if it becomes necessary.

Step 4 – The analytical phase

Once data is collected, analysis is undertaken. Collation of the results, where individual participant results are transferred to the appropriate data analysis package, can be undertaken as the study progresses, with the appropriate consideration of secure storage, the Data Protection Act, participant anonymity and confidentiality. The analysis method should have been designed with the assistance of statistical advice. Statistical analysis methods are considered in Chapter 5.

The research process should also be analysed. The research experience should be compared to the original plan and any strengths or weakness identified, along with the potential impact on the research findings. With most studies, something goes awry – study participants withdraw in greater numbers than expected, the data collector is sick, or one of the team invents a 'new way', which could impact on the findings. This is very frustrating, but realistically these problems are as much a part of research as they are of clinical practice. It is important to document such issues, as they can contribute to the planning of subsequent studies and may directly help practice issues. In reports this aspect of the analysis is usually within the discussion section.

Step 5 – The dissemination phase

The final stage of the research process, which is an important responsibility of all researchers, is to make known the findings from their study. This involves the publication not just of the research findings but also of information about the research process. This publication may be through journals, local and national conferences or through personal networking. If midwifery practice is to become evidence-based then it is important that research is made public. It is then the responsibility of all practitioners to take the time to read the information, critique and apply it as appropriate to their practice, the skills for which are explored in Chapter 10.

Answers to questions about hypothesis and variables, Box 3.2

The null hypotheses would be:
- There is no difference in pain experience or pethidine use between women using aromatherapy and those who do not
- The use of tea bags makes no difference to nipple pain in breastfeeding women
- There is no difference in midwives' knowledge and skills whether or not they attend five study days.

Please note that the null hypothesis can be worded in several ways, so if your version is different but still indicates no difference then you are correct.

Research variables
In each of the above statements the independent variables are:
aromatherapy, tea bags, five study days.

In each of the above statements the dependent variables are:
pain experience and pethidine use, nipple pain, midwives' knowledge and skills.

CONCLUSION

The key to a good experimental research study is a logical and carefully constructed plan that takes into account the needs of both the clinical setting and the research process. This is evident in this chapter by the proportion of space that has been devoted to step 2. Then the plan must be carried out, with constant attention to detail and the documentation of all stages. Researchers need to be vigilant, conscientious and committed to their work. Midwives have much to offer experimental research and it has much to offer midwifery; the art is in recognizing both the topics and the midwives who have the potential to use the experimental research process to the benefit of women and their children.

CHAPTER SUMMARY

This chapter has highlighted that:
The quantitative research process can be considered in five steps:

Step 1 – Formulate a precise research question, including reviewing the literature

Step 2 – Plan the study in detail, including ethics approval

Step 3 – Collect the data – the empirical phase

Step 4 – Analyse the data

Step 5 – Tell the world your results – dissemination

The main quantitative research designs are:

◆ Experimental research including randomized controlled studies, such as:
   - Post-test-only studies
   - Pre- and post-test studies
   - Solomon Four designs
   - Factorial designs

◆ Matched pair design

◆ Quasi-experimental designs, including:
   - Nonequivalent groups
   - Time series designs
   - Ex post facto designs
   - One-group-only designs

◆ Experimental case studies

For high quality quantitative studies remember:

To consider the measurement tool used

To consider intra- and inter-rater variability

You must pilot all aspects of the research process

REFERENCES

Alexander J 1996 The Southampton randomized controlled trial of breast shells and Hoffman's exercises for inverted and non-protractile nipples. In: Robinson S, Thomson A M (ed) Midwives, research and childbirth, vol 4. Chapman & Hall, London, ch 8, p 165–191

Ayres J 1995 Midwifery literature: getting started. Modern Midwife 5(11): 27–28

Baum M 1993 New approach for the recruitment into randomized control trials. Lancet 341: 812–813

Brewin C R, Bradley C 1989 Patient preference and randomized clinical trials. British Medical Journal 299: 313–315

Burns N, Grove S K 1993 The practice of nursing research. Conduct, critique and utilisation, 2nd edn. WB Saunders, Philadelphia, PA, ch 7, p 141–164

Chalmers I, Enkin M, Keirse M J N C (ed) 1989 Effective care in pregnancy and childbirth, vols 1 and 2. Oxford University Press, Oxford

Cluett ER, Alexander J, Pickering R M 1995 Is measuring the postnatal symphysis–fundal distance worthwhile? Midwifery 11(4): 174–183

Collier J 1995 Confusion over the use of placebos in clinical trials. British Medical Journal 311: 821–822

Cook T D, Campbell D T 1979 Quasi experimentation: design and analysis issues for field settings. Rand McNally, College Publishing Company, USA

Dawson J 1986 Randomized trials and informed consent in neonatal medicine. British Medical Journal 296: 1373–1374

Department of Health 1991 Health service guidelines. Local ethics committees. HMSO, London

Department of Health 1992 Assessing the effects of health technologies: principles, practice, proposals. Department of Health. HMSO, London

Drayton S, Rees C 1989 Is anyone out there still giving enemas? In: Robinson S, Thomson AM (ed) Midwives, research and childbirth. vol 1. Chapman & Hall, London, ch 7, p 139–154

Ernst E, Resch K L 1995 Concept of true and perceived placebo effect. British Medical Journal. 311: 551–553

Gallo C, Perrone F, De Placido S, Giusti C 1995 Informed versus randomized consent to clinical trials. Lancet 364: 1060–1064

Greenwood J 1984 Nursing research: a position paper. Journal of Advanced Nursing 9: 77–82

Hawkins S 1997 Databases. Modern Midwife 7(1): 27–28

Johnson A 1997 Randomized controlled trials in perinatal medicine: 3. Identifying and measuring endpoints in randomized controlled trials. British Journal of Obstetrics and Gynaecology 104(7): 768–771

Keeble S 1995 Experimental research 1. An introduction to experimental design. Open Learning Foundation. Churchill Livingstone, Edinburgh

Kennell J, Klaus M, McGarth S, Robertson S, Hinkley C 1991 Continuous emotional support during labour in a US hospital. A randomized controlled trial. Journal of the American Medical Association 265(17): 2197–2201

Meinert C L, Tonascia S 1986 Clinical trials. Design, conduct and analysis. Oxford University Press, Oxford

Moore W, James D R 1989 A random trial of three topical analgesic agents in the treatment of episiotomy pain following instrumental delivery. Journal of Obstetrics and Gynaecology 10(1): 35–39

Oakley A 1990 Cause or causation? – The role of random numbers. Women and Health 15(4): 31–42

ORACLE Clinical Coordinating Centre 1996 ORACLE. MRC Preterm antibiotic uncertainty study. Protocol, 2nd ed. ORACLE Clinical Co-ordinating Centre, Leicester

Parahoo A K 1997 Nursing research. Principles, process and issues. Macmillan, Basingstoke

Parmar M K B 1992 Randomization before consent: practical and ethical considerations. In: Williams C J (ed) Introducing new treatments for cancer. Practical, ethical and legal problems. John Wiley, Chichester, ch 14, p 189–201

Pocock S J 1983 Clinical trial. A practical approach. John Wiley, Chichester

Polit D F, Hungler B P 1997 Essentials of nursing research. Methods appraisal and utilization, 4th edn. JB Lippincott, Philadelphia, PA

Prendiville W, Harding J, Elbourne D, Stirrat G 1988 The Bristol third stage trial: active versus physiological management of the third stage of labour. British Medical Journal 297: 1295–3000

Ramler D, Roberts J 1986 A comparison of cold and warm sitz baths for relief of postpartum perineal pain. Journal of Obstetric, Gynaecologic and Neonatal Nursing 15: 471–474

Rees C 1997 An introduction to research for midwives. Books for Midwives Press, Cheshire

Reid N 1993 Health care research by degrees. Blackwell Scientific, Oxford

Roethlisberger F J, Dickson W J 1939 Management and the worker. Harvard University Press, Cambridge, MA

Romney M L, Gordon H 1981 Is your enema really necessary? British Medical Journal 282: 1269–1271

Sapsford R, Abbott P 1992 Research methods for nurses and the caring professions. Open University Press, Buckingham

Schwartz D, Lellouch J 1967 Explanatory and pragmatic attitudes in therapeutic trials. Journal of Chronic Disease 20: 637–648

Silverman W A 1994 Patients' preferences and randomized trials. Lancet 343: 1586

Sleep J M 1990 Postnatal perineal care. In: Alexander J, Levy V, Roch S (ed) Postnatal care: a research based approach. Macmillan, Basingstoke, ch 1, p 1–17

Sleep J M, Grant A 1987 Pelvic exercises in postnatal care – the report of a randomized controlled trial to compare an intensive exercise regimen with the programme in current use. Midwifery 3: 158–164

Sleep J M, Grant A 1988 Routine addition of salt or Savlon bath concentrate during bathing in the immediate post-partum period. A randomized controlled trial. Nursing Times 84(21): 55–57

Toth B 1997 Web brings Medline to the desktop and it can be free. Evidence based purchasing. R & D Directorate. NHS Executive South and West 18(July): 1

Wilson-Barnett J 1991 The experiment: is it worth it? International Journal of Nursing Studies 28(1): 77–87

World Medical Association 1989 Declaration of Helsinki. Recommendations guiding physicians in biomedical research involving human subjects. Adopted 1964, updated last September 1989 at the 41st World Medical Assembly, Hong Kong

Zelen M 1979 A new design for randomized clinical trials. New England Journal of Medicine 300(22): 1242–1245

Zelen M 1990 Randomized consent designs for clinical trials: an update. Statistics in Medicine 9: 645–656

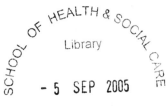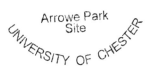

Surveys

Pam Wagstaff

KEY ISSUES

- ◆ The purpose of surveys
- ◆ Methods and tools used within surveys
- ◆ Questionnaires
- ◆ Scales
- ◆ Interviews
- ◆ Components of the survey approach
- ◆ Reliability and validity
- ◆ The Delphi Survey

INTRODUCTION

The survey approach is **quantitative** and **nonexperimental** because it does not involve the manipulation of variables. The term survey is used in two different ways in relation to research. It can be defined as research that aims to obtain descriptive and/or **correlational** data using questionnaires, interviews and occasionally observation. This means that, while surveys can identify relationships between the variables under study, they cannot determine whether that relationship is **causal** or not. The inability to consider causality is what distinguishes surveys from the **experimental** approach. Alternatively, survey can refer to any research based on **probability sampling**. Generally the analysis of data is statistical in order to describe or model the characteristics of the population under study or to answer research questions (Czaja and Blair 1996). Surveys should only be used when several simple but essential conditions are met: the target population is clearly defined; the target population is easily identified; and the majority of the respondents will be able to answer the questions asked. In this chapter the first definition of surveys has been adopted and I will focus on survey designs and the principal tools used within this approach, i.e. questionnaires and structured interviews.

PURPOSE

Surveys are normally undertaken to collect information about a well-defined population. The information that can be collected is diverse but essentially is related to the prevalence, distribution and inter-relationships of variables (Polit and Hungler 1995). The aim is not to discover the cause of phenomena but to produce accurate quantitative descriptions (Treece and Treece 1986). Data collected is varied and includes demographic information, what people do, how they behave and what they believe, feel or think. Data collection techniques normally used are questionnaire, face-to-face interviews and telephone interviews (Fink and Kosecoff 1985), with data being collected over days, weeks, months or even several years (Robinson and Owen 1994). Observation can also be used to obtain data (Parahoo 1997). Surveys can therefore generate knowledge about maternity services and midwifery practice in order to improve the quality of care provided. Like any other form of research, the purpose of surveys has to be for the benefit of those being studied and not for the benefit of the researcher (Wagstaff 1998, Robinson 1996).

Audits, for example the Confidential Enquiries into Stillbirths and Deaths in Infancy (Wessex Institute 1997), use the same types of data collection method, particularly demographic and clinical data. The Audit Commission (Garcia et al 1998) surveyed women's views of maternity care and provided useful data on women's experiences and feelings.

CHARACTERISTICS OF THE APPROACH

Advantages of surveys

The main advantage of the survey technique is the relative ease of recruiting a large sample and obtaining data at relatively low cost. A broad range of phenomena can be studied, providing insight into aspects of care provision including attitudes, values, beliefs and behaviours. This may subsequently lead to the development of other research questions. Survey techniques can be used for almost any known population with a high degree of generalizability. As a result of their structured nature, the data are amenable to statistical analysis. As a result of these two facets, survey findings are considered to be objective (Smith 1975, Treece and Treece 1986, Mitchell and Jolley 1996).

Disadvantages of surveys

This research approach is dependent on the motivation and ability of respondents to reply truthfully. Surveys are open to memory or viewpoint bias and the questionnaire or interview may lack validity. There is very little control over extraneous variables.

COMPONENTS OF THE RESEARCH PROCESS

The research process associated with the survey approach is shown in Fig. 4.1 and each component is then discussed.

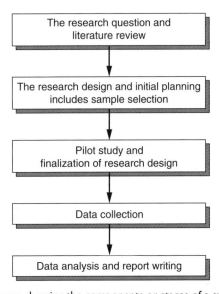

Figure 4.1 Flow diagram showing the components or stages of a survey

The research question and literature review

Researchers must clarify what they wish to investigate and why. This clarification involves a literature review, which identifies what is known and helps in the design of the research study by, for example, identifying tools that are already available and problems that other researchers have encountered. The researchers will be able to clarify the aims and objectives of their survey. A decision can then be made about whether the survey will be descriptive and/or correlational. This will be expressed in either a research question or a hypothesis.

The research design and initial planning

The best way to collect data and which research tools to use will be determined by the purpose of the research study. The quality and depth of the data that is required and an awareness of the strengths and weaknesses of the different data collection techniques will also inform the design. Every effort should be made to make the survey as good as it can be. However, Sudman (1976) suggests that researchers should consider how good the survey needs to be, this being linked to the purpose of the survey. Consideration needs to be given to obtaining ethical approval where necessary. As with any form of research, poorly designed studies are unethical as they involve the use of clients and/or staff without adding to the body of knowledge. Even completing a short questionnaire involves someone's time and effort.

Sample

The target population for the study needs to be clearly defined. The sample size and method of selection can then be determined. The sampling frame, i.e. the eligible population from which the sample can be selected, can then be found or developed. Although **convenience sampling** is often used for practical reasons, **random** or **probability sampling**, where every member of the population has a known chance of being selected is preferable. It may also be of value to use either a **stratified** or a **quota sample** to ensure that the sample is representative. Proud and Murphy-Black (1997) used a stratified sample to ensure that all types of maternity unit were included in their survey on the amount of information given to women who were deciding whether to have an ultrasound scan.

There is no simple answer as to how large the sample should be: generally the bigger the better. A detailed explanation of the complex mathematical procedures used to determine sample size, i.e. **power calculations**, is given in Czaja and Blair 1996. In practice, the sampling method will depend on the researchers' knowledge of the population and the resources available. Bick and MacArthur (1995) had to exclude Asian women from their survey relating to postnatal examinations, as the study included a follow-up interview and there were no resources available to employ an interpreter. In situations such as this, researchers and those reading the published paper must consider how such exclusions affect the representativeness of the sample and therefore the ability to generalize the findings. Ethical issues also need to be considered when selecting the sample; for example, Robinson (1996) warns of the distress and anxiety that can be caused when women with sick children are questioned about smoking in pregnancy.

Pilot study and finalization of the design

It is important that the research design is pretested. Bell (1987) suggests that those responding to a pilot questionnaire are asked:

◆ Were the instructions clear?
◆ How long did it take to complete?
◆ Were the questions ambiguous?
◆ Did you object to any questions, and if so, why?
◆ Do you think any topic area has been omitted?

This piloting will identify problems with the design or research tools that can be rectified before the main study begins. Changes may be required after piloting the various aspects of the study. If extensive alterations are made a second pilot should be conducted.

Data collection

The period of data collection will vary depending on the design of the survey and the research tools being used. Researchers should have a realistic timescale. During data collection there must be meticulous attention to detail and careful organization to ensure that the design is followed consistently throughout the research period.

Data analysis and report writing

Data analysis should be considered at the planning stage. The method used will depend on the size of the survey and the facilities available. Coding is the process whereby responses are classified so the data can be analysed by a computer statistical package such as SPSS (Norusis 1990) or by hand. With a small sample it may be possible to analyse data without coding. However, for most surveys coding is necessary and this is relatively simple to carry out. Some researchers incorporate codes at the side of the questionnaire.

With closed questions, coding is relatively easy: for example, if the choice of answer is Yes or No, 'Yes' is given the code 1 and 'No' the code 2. Similarly, if there is a choice of six responses, they can be coded from 1 to 6. Data can then be loaded on to a computer for analysis using descriptive and/or inferential statistics. Open questions are more difficult to analyse. It may be possible to categorize responses or identify themes. Responses may be used verbatim to add depth to the quantitative analyses. There are potential dangers in collating the qualitative data rather than analysing it, or paying little attention to it in the final results. Further information on coding, analyses and presentation of data is available in Bell 1987, Mitchell and Jolley 1996, Blaxter et al 1996, Jowett and Shanley 1993 and Oppenheim 1992.

SPECIFIC TOOLS AND METHODS WITHIN THE APPROACH

The questionnaire

A questionnaire is a set of standard questions that the respondent answers unaided. Questions can be related to knowledge, behaviour, attitudes, opinions or beliefs (Sudman and Bradburn 1982). Surveys using questionnaires are a popular way of collecting information because they can be obtained with a minimum amount of time and expense and can cover a large geographical area. Data collected may, however, lack depth and there is no opportunity to observe nonverbal cues. Overuse of questionnaires can mean that respondents are 'fed up' with being asked to complete them. It is therefore vital that care is taken in the design of the questionnaire and its administration. Respondents need to be clear about the purpose of the study and how the information is going to be used so that they feel their contribution is valued.

Questionnaire development

A good questionnaire is one that is constructed in such a way that the appropriate information is obtained. Through the process of reviewing the literature or talking to experts, the researchers may gain information on how to develop their own questionnaire or identify an existing one that will meet their needs. The Office of Population Censuses and Surveys (OPCS) developed a survey manual (Mason 1989) to help health authorities monitor the views of maternity services users. This manual gives a step-by-step guide to the assessment of women's views and includes pretested questionnaires. The validity and reliability of established questionnaires must not be assumed. This is particularly important if the questionnaire was designed and tested in a different country or for a different subject group.

To maintain the interest and motivation of respondents, thought should go into its construction and administration. The questionnaire should be well presented: this includes neatness, readability, accurate spelling and the use of good-quality paper. Long questions should be avoided. Oppenheim (1992) suggests no more than 20 words. Consideration needs to be given to the length of the questionnaire: if it is too long respondents can be deterred from completing or even starting it. Treece and Treece (1986) suggest that questionnaires should not normally take longer than 20–25 minutes to complete. However, a longer questionnaire may be appropriate if the respondent has an intrinsic interest in its subject matter and believes it is important.

Language and terminology should be appropriate for the anticipated respondents. If they do not understand the questions, they may not respond or their response may be a guess. This affects the response rate and the reliability and validity of data collected. To help respondents feel comfortable, questionnaires should start with easy questions. Questions should move from the general to the specific. They should be arranged so they flow and fit in with the respondents' thought processes. If the structure of the questionnaire makes sense to respondents it is more likely that they will remain interested and complete it.

It is generally agreed that personal and/or sensitive questions such as those relating to age, marital status and income should be at the end of the questionnaire, with a clear rationale for their inclusion. Williamson and Thomson (1996) identified problems with the collection of such demographic data while piloting a questionnaire to determine women's satisfaction with antenatal care. Women objected to the question 'Do you live rent-free?' To avoid a poor response rate, particularly from women in lower socioeconomic groups this question was removed. However some sensitive questions may be necessary to achieve the research aims: a balance is needed.

If the response is to be returned by post, questionnaires should be accompanied by a stamped, self-addressed envelope to reduce costs to respondents. If you are using questionnaires that respondents are asked to complete at a certain time, e.g. when attending an antenatal clinic (Williamson and Thomson 1996), there should be sufficient pens available, with extras in case they disappear. There should be clear instructions as to where the questionnaire should be left or to whom it should be handed.

Types of question

One of the keys to a good questionnaire is asking the right questions in the right way; this framing of questions does take time and practice. Czaja and Blair (1996) warn that many drafts of a questionnaire may be necessary before it is right. One of the first decisions is whether to use open or closed questions or scales or a combination.

Closed questions give the respondent a limited choice of answers, which may be Yes or No or a choice from a selection of responses. It is generally easier to analyse closed questions, but they may give little insight into the research question. A closed question could be:

Were you satisfied with the care you received in labour?   Yes/No

Open questions allow respondents to answer in their own words. This allows expression of feelings, values and beliefs. They do, however, put an extra burden on respondents, particularly if they are not articulate or have limited writing skills (McColl 1993). Open questions are more difficult and time-consuming to analyse. Questions can be devised for a narrow or broad response. For example a question requiring a narrow response could be:

List the three main aspects of care in labour you were satisfied and dis-satisfied with.

Satisfied

1 ————————————

2 ————————————

3 ————————————

Dissatisfied

1 ————————————

2 ————————————

3 ————————————

A broader response could be obtained by asking:

What is your opinion of the care you received in labour?

————————————————————————

————————————————————————

————————————————————————

The amount the respondent writes will depend on the space available, which suggests what is expected. Providing respondents with the opportunity to be expansive does not mean that they will be. For example, the response to the last question could be as little as 'OK'.

When designing questions some common problems should be avoided (Box 4.1).

Scales

Scales are a useful way of collecting standardized measurable data relating to certain characteristics or behaviour. Data collected can readily be manipulated, analysed and interpreted. The use of scales produces a single score indicating the direction and intensity of respondents' attitudes. These scales can take several forms and those discussed in this chapter are the Likert scale, semantic differential scale, visual analogue scale and Guttman or cumulative scale.

Likert scale

The Likert scale is one of the best known types of scale and is commonly used to measure attitudes (Box 4.2).

It requires the respondent to select, from a small number of ordered alternatives, their attitude to a particular statement. There is some disagreement in the literature as to whether the Likert scale yields **ordinal** (Oppenheim

Box 4.1 Common problems with questionnaire questions

◆ **Ambiguity:** use language that has the same meaning for everybody

◆ **Biased or leading questions** that suggest the answer expected, e.g. 'Do you believe, like most informed midwives, that women should be allowed a home delivery if they want one?'

◆ **Hypothetical questions** such as:
'How would you respond to...?'
We cannot always tell how we would respond in certain situations. We can only comment on how we think we would respond or how we would like to think we would respond. A more accurate and valid response is likely from the question:
'How did you respond to...?'

◆ **Double negatives**, as the response required is not clear, e.g. 'Are you against not allowing midwives to top up epidurals?'

◆ When restricting the response to a set of given statements, called 'forced responses', **ensure the list is comprehensive**. If this is not done, there may be no response or one that is invalid, as it does not reflect the respondent's views.

◆ **Multiple questions** such as:
'Do women get enough support antenatally, during labour, and postnatally?   YES/NO'
The answer may be Yes for one part of the question but not for others.

◆ If a questionnaire is to be translated for subjects for whom English is not the first language care should be taken that **the original meaning of questions is not lost in translation**. To achieve this, Holroyd et al (1997) first translated an English language questionnaire into Chinese and then had the Chinese version translated back into English by an independent bilingual midwife. A second bilingual midwife compared these translated versions to ensure that the meaning of the questions remained the same.

1992) or **interval** data (Mitchell and Jolley 1996). Ordinal implies that the distance or degree of change between two adjacent statements is different from that between other statements on the scale. Interval data implies that the distance or degree of change between all the statements is identical. Rensis Likert, the psychologist, originally used five alternatives:

strongly agree, agree, uncertain, disagree, strongly disagree.

Other researchers use seven alternatives adding 'slightly agree' and 'slightly

---

Box 4.2 Example of a Likert scale

◆ **Women should be able to choose their place of confinement**
Strongly agree/Agree/Uncertain/Disagree/Strongly disagree

◆ **How helpful was the advice given to you by your midwife?**
Very helpful/Helpful/No comment/Not helpful/Very unhelpful

---

disagree'. This allows for respondents who do not have strong views or have not made up their mind on the subject (Polit and Hungler 1995).

To avoid introducing bias there should be an equal number of positive and negative responses. Responses are scored so that agreement with positively worded statements and nonagreement with negatively worded statements are awarded higher scores. The scores are added up and analysed. Only responses to questions relating to the same concept should be scored together. If the topic has a number of different dimensions these should be scored separately. Careful consideration has to be given to the questions used to ensure that they can discriminate between the different topic dimensions. Questions can be developed from a previous exploratory study on the subject. Hicks (1995) reduced 38 statements to 13 by ensuring that only discriminating questions were used.

Semantic differential scale

Semantic differential scales are highly flexible, easily constructed scales used to rate a specific concept, e.g. an individual, a situation, a service or more abstract concepts. They are based on the ability of language to reflect a person's feelings. The questions or statements require a response between conflicting adjectives (Howe 1995). Bipolar rating scales such as Satisfied/Unsatisfied, Pleasant/Unpleasant specify the two ends of a continuum allowing the respondent to indicate where on this continuum their views fit. A scale of 7 is most commonly used but this can be reduced to 5 or increased to 9. For example, women could be asked their views of those involved in their care using the scales in Fig. 4.2.

Scoring of responses is similar to that for Likert scales. In this example the scale would be scored from 1–7; the values are not however printed on the form. The position of the positive adjective should be varied as this is more likely to ensure that the choices are read and the respondent does not pick one point in the scale and tick down. In the example in Fig. 4.2, competent scores 7 and incompetent scores 1, while rude scores 1 and polite scores 7.

Question: How would you rate the midwife who cared for you during delivery?

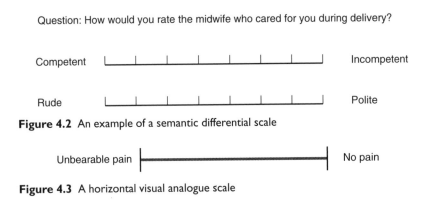

Competent Incompetent

Rude Polite

Figure 4.2 An example of a semantic differential scale

Unbearable pain No pain

Figure 4.3 A horizontal visual analogue scale

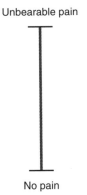

Unbearable pain

No pain

Figure 4.4 A vertical visual analogue scale

Visual analogue scale

The visual analogue scale (VAS) is similar to the semantic differential but, instead of identified gradations on the scale, there is normally a 100 mm straight line with the extremes of responses to the phenomenon at each end (Cline et al 1992). Responses can be recorded anywhere on the line. The scale may lie in a horizontal or vertical direction, with the lowest end of the scale being on the left of the horizontal line or at the bottom of the vertical line (Figs 4.3 and 4.4; Gift 1989).

Benefits of the visual analogue scale include its simplicity and the ease with which it can be administered and completed. It is also useful when measuring changes over time. For these reasons it is commonly used in research and practice to measure subjective feelings such as anxiety, attitudes and perceptions, as well as physiological symptoms such as pain and nausea.

Guttman or cumulative scales

The Guttman or cumulative scale was developed by Louis Guttman and his associates during the 1940s and contains a set of items with which the respondent agrees or disagrees. Items should relate to only one concept and should be designed in such a way that they are presented in a hierarchy. In the example below, if women in preterm labour visiting the neonatal unit (NNU) agree with item 3 they should also agree with statements 1 and 2. If they agree with statement 5 they should agree with statements 1–5. The score given to the respondent equals the number of responses she agreed with (Box 4.3).

Box 4.3 An example of a Guttman scale box

1. Women at risk of a preterm delivery should have the opportunity of visiting the NNU.

2. Women at risk of preterm delivery should be informed that they can visit the NNU.

3. Women at risk of preterm delivery should be told of the benefits of visiting the NNU.

4. Women at risk of preterm delivery should be actively encouraged to visit the NNU.

5. Every women at risk of preterm delivery should be taken on a visit to the NNU.

Further information on these scales is available in Oppenheim 1992, Priest et al 1995, Howe 1995, Cline et al 1992, Lee and Kieckhefer 1989, Sudman and Bradurn 1982 and Miller 1991.

Distribution of questionnaires and cover letters

Questionnaires can be postal or handed directly to respondents. Postal surveys may use internal hospital or public systems. Additionally, questionnaires may be sent to a named person, such as a senior sister, for distribution. Postal surveys save time and effort for the researcher. However, it is not known if the questionnaires have been received, or whether they were completed by the person intended. These problems do not usually occur when a questionnaire is given to an individual personally, however Williamson and Thomson (1996) describe how young women in an antenatal clinic frequently gave a self-administered patient satisfaction questionnaire to their mothers to complete despite being asked to complete the questionnaires themselves. Personal distribution is time-consuming and only possible in a small geographical area such as the researchers' own unit.

A cover letter is essential for most surveys using questionnaires, although it may not be necessary where the researcher has distributed and explained the questionnaire in person. The cover letter should explain the purpose of the research and who is supporting it. If ethical approval has been granted it is advisable to state this. It should give clear instructions on how the questionnaire should be completed, how and to whom the questionnaire should be returned, and by what date. In determining when questionnaires should be returned you should consider how long it will take to reach respondents and whether potential respondents might be on holiday. An explanation of what will happen to the data and assurances of anonymity and confidentiality should be included. It should be clear to respondents why their participation is important and they should be thanked for their time and effort. Signing each letter gives them a personal feel.

Before the questionnaire and cover letter are distributed it may be appropriate to contact those in the sample, as Meldrum et al (1994) did when surveying the understanding of terminology relating to maternity services. Those in the sample were initially contacted by telephone and informed about the purpose of the study. Of 22 questionnaires sent, 21 were returned. This study involved a very small sample and contacting individuals may not be feasible when the sample size is large. Direct contact may be time-consuming and expensive. Midwives on limited budgets may not be able to achieve this.

Response rate

There is no clear definition of what is an acceptable response rate. Miller (1991) suggests that response rates to postal questionnaires are typically low, quoting a figure of 50% if conducted by a relatively inexperienced person. Treece and Treece (1986) suggest that a response rate of 75–85% from a postal survey is very good. The response rate for postal surveys will depend on the accuracy of the postal list. Bick and MacArthur (1995), in a survey relating to postnatal health, had 61 of 1667 questionnaires returned by the Post Office for women no longer at the given address. As a result, they calculated their response rate on the number of questionnaires believed to have been correctly delivered, i.e. 1606.

It is important to know as much as possible about nonresponders, as those who do not respond may differ from those who do (Moser and Kalton 1971), and so introduce bias in the sampling. Robinson and Owen (1994), for example, identified that in the second stage of their survey nonpractising midwives were under-represented among the respondents. There is, however, an ethical issue relating to the collection of information about nonresponders, who by declining to participate have not given their consent for the use of their data.

Dillman (1978) suggests that response rates will be higher if the cost to the respondent in terms of time and effort is minimal and the reward is maximal. Rewards can include intangible aspects such as feeling useful, being appreciated and positive regard, which can be expressed in the cover letter or through personalized contact (Crosby et al 1989).

The largest proportion of returns are likely to occur within the first few days, with fewer responses likely as time passes. To increase the rate of response, some form of follow-up can be useful such as a letter reminding respondents of the questionnaire and possibly including a further copy. This has been shown to increase responses by 20% on average (Miller 1991), with second and third follow-up mailings showing an additional 12% and 10% response respectively. There are, however, wide variations. Pretesting the distribution and return of questionnaires may help in determining how much time should be left before such follow-up occurs.

If researchers cannot tell who has returned questionnaires it will be necessary to circulate follow-up correspondence to the whole sample. This increases researchers' workload and may annoy those who have already returned their questionnaires. Many researchers code either the questionnaire or the self-addressed envelope in some way, such as numbering them, so that they can identify respondents. This should not affect anonymity, as the researcher should make no further link between the responses and the respondent.

Various methods have been tried to maximize the response to questionnaires (Box 4.4).

Box 4.4 An example of how one group of researchers maximized their response rates

In a study of the careers of various cohorts of newly qualified midwives, Robinson and Owen (1994) tried to maximize their response rate by:

◆ piloting their questionnaire

◆ ensuring validity and reliability

◆ ensuring acceptability to respondents

◆ checking the reliability of respondents' addresses

◆ sending short feedback reports to respondents to maintain their interest

◆ sending reminder letters and duplicate questionnaires

◆ asking those who did respond to contact any members of their cohort who did not.

Interviews

Face-to-face interviews

Interviews are popular tools for collecting survey information. The structured interview is generally used in surveys. Each question is asked in the same order and format, with no variation. The design of the interview is very much like that of a questionnaire. The interviewer asks questions in the order specified, recording responses or even coding the responses as the interview proceeds. Closed questions are most commonly used; however, unlike questionnaires, the interviewer can clarify and further explain questions to the respondent. The interviewer may also observe nonverbal cues, which may indicate when the respondent has not understood something. The interviewer should remember that the aim of a structured interview is to achieve standardization, so the same information should be available to all respondents (Parahoo 1997). In the presence of an interviewer, responses are more likely to be honest than they would be if respondents completed the questionnaire (Newell 1994). However, it could be argued that having an interviewer present increases the risk of interview bias. The structured interview has similar advantages to questionnaires in that responses can be compared across samples and populations and statistical analyses of responses is relatively easy. Because the format is so structured, any variation in response cannot be considered to be due to the way the questionnaire is administered.

Disadvantages of the structured interview are similar to those of the questionnaire. There is a lack of depth, because of the type of question asked, and a reduced ability to expand on the subject. Interviews are more time-consuming and expensive and interviewer bias can be introduced, with the interviewer in some way influencing the respondent's responses. Respondents are more likely to give socially desirable answers than they would if responding to an anonymous questionnaire (Mitchell and Jolley 1996).

Telephone interviews

This is an increasingly used tool for data collection in social sciences, because of the increasing percentage of the population who have a telephone. A wide geographical area can be reached, and it is cheaper than personal interviews. Miller (1991) suggests that in America the cost can be reduced to 45–65% of the costs of the personal interview. It is also less costly in terms of time involvement for the interviewer. It has been suggested that researchers only spend approximately one-third of their time in undertaking a face-to-face interview, the rest of the time is used in travel and finding respondents (Oppenheim 1992). The telephone interview can normally be completed in a short time, which may be advantageous to both researcher and respondent.

Additionally, respondents may feel more at ease answering sensitive questions than in a face-to-face interview. Conversely, Miller (1991) suggests that there is likely to be less rapport between the interviewer and the respondent, making it less rewarding. This may explain lower response rates than in personal interviews. Silences during the conversation can be uncomfortable for the respondent, and the interviewer cannot read or respond to body language.

Telephone interviews are more costly in terms of time and effort for the researcher than postal surveys. They may not be the best method if the respondent needs to refer to sources of information in order to answer a question. The type of question asked can be affected by the respondents' ability to retain information, so questions need to be short and relatively simple: no more than 20 words. If the respondent has choices between responses these should be few in number, short and simple: if too many are given the respondent may only remember the first or last and so potential bias is introduced (Czaja and Blair 1996).

A potential disadvantage of this technique is that the sample may not be representative, as respondents have to possess a telephone. Lack of access to a telephone is associated more with being in a lower-income family, being young and male and having recently moved house (Oppenheim 1992). Access to telephone numbers via the phone book can be problematic as more people go ex-directory. Midwives may generate their sampling frame from case notes that include contact numbers.

Czaja and Blair (1996) suggest that the telephone interview may be an appropriate survey technique when attitudinal and behavioural questions are asked, as these can be answered from memory. The interview should not last longer than 30 minutes. Consideration needs to be given to the time of day at which the interview will take place, as this needs to suit the respondent. This can be decided through direct contact with potential subjects, by letter or preliminary phone call. An unplanned phone call is likely to result in a high refusal rate.

The Delphi technique

The Delphi technique is a survey method used for obtaining judgements, predictions or opinions from a panel of experts through structured communication. It differs from other survey methods in that it is iterative: this involves the use of a series of self-report questionnaires interspersed with controlled feedback of results to the participants. Subsequent questionnaires are developed from responses to the previous one, in an attempt to achieve group consensus (Fig. 4.5).

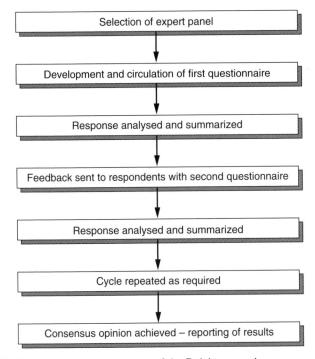

Figure 4.5 Diagrammatic representation of the Delphi research process

Origins and purpose

This survey method was developed in the early 1950s by the RAND Corporation in the US and it is used for obtaining the most reliable consensus of expert opinion on a topic when face-to-face meetings are not feasible and/or desirable. This research method takes its name from Delphi, the site of a temple complex in ancient Greece where a priestess made prophesies about the future (Everett 1993). It was designed for long-range forecasting of trends, particularly in relation to science and technology, and their impact on society.

Linstone and Turoff (1975), editors of the seminal work on the Delphi technique, suggest that it is an appropriate method to use when the research question is not readily answered by purely analytical techniques. It has been used to determine the characteristics of optimum practice (Butterworth 1995) and for clinical research priorities (Bond and Bond 1982). Although the Delphi technique was originally devised to ascertain a consensus view of experts, Procter and Hunt (1994) suggest that it could be used to highlight divergence and contradictions.

Advantages and disadvantages of Delphi surveys

The key advantage is the structured group communication between individuals on complex, broad or uncertain issues, even though the group may be geographically separated. The effect of interpersonal feelings and actions that can influence the findings of the group are removed, with each expert's response being given equal value. Anonymity can be assured, so participants should be able to give their true opinions and be fully involved throughout the process. Feedback aids this sense of participation. As a consensus view is usually achieved, Delphi surveys demonstrate the state of informed opinion at the time of the research (McKenna 1994). The process can be expensive in terms of money and time in recruiting experts, devising questionnaires and summarizing responses, as well as the cost of printing and circulating questionnaires. A large quantity of data requiring analysis can be generated, particularly if a qualitative approach towards data is taken. The process can also be lengthy and dependent on respondents returning questionnaires within a reasonable time frame, and poor responses have been reported for later rounds of the process (Strachan 1996, McKenna 1994).

The selection of a panel of experts is based on their knowledge of the field of study. It is important to ensure that those selected are representative of the field, for the findings to be valid (Goodman 1987) and accepted by others. The structure and organization of the initial questionnaire is important, as this will determine subsequent responses (Procter and Hunt 1994). The questionnaire can use open or closed questions. It may ask respondents to create lists, or may consist of statements to which a response is required. Researchers collate and summarize the information collected. Feedback to respondents is given in the form of a summary of the results together with a new questionnaire. This process is repeated, usually up to a maximum of four times, until there is a general consensus of opinions, beliefs or predictions from the experts.

RELIABILITY AND VALIDITY

Reliability and validity must be considered in relation to the complete survey design as well as to specific questions used. Reliability is the consistency with which a tool can measure what it intended to measure, in the given environment. Four factors related to reliability or response error in surveys are memory, motivation, communication and knowledge (Sudman and Bradburn 1982). Memory is not always reliable. Respondents may be motivated to reply in a certain way, such as giving acquiescent responses, or may lack motivation and respond inappropriately. They may not understand the question or may lack the knowledge to answer. Occasionally, someone other than the targeted respondent may answer the survey. This is most likely with questionnaires, where its completion may be delegated to a junior.

One simple way of determining reliability is the test–retest process. Individuals are asked to complete the questionnaire and to repeat the process a few weeks later. Responses should be the same unless something has happened to change the respondent's knowledge, views or attitudes. An alternate-form or equivalence test could be used, when the same question is asked in a different way within the questionnaire. There are specific statistical tests to analyse this type of reliability testing.

Validity is to do with the notion of truth, that is you are measuring what you think you are measuring. Validity can be considered in several ways and includes **content validity**, **criterion-related validity** and **construct validity**. Each of these can used to test the validity of surveys, as well as other forms of quantitative research.

Content validity is the degree to which the questionnaire encompasses and represents what is being studied and is particularly important for questionnaires designed to measure knowledge or attitudes. It involves an assessment of whether the questionnaire includes everything it should. Polit and Hungler (1995) suggest that there is no completely objective way of assuring content validity as it will be determined by other people's judgements, such as those of experts or a panel of judges with experience of the subject area.

Criterion-related validity is about how well the survey performs in relation to other already validated measures of the same subject area. Data from the new survey is compared with data collected by the other measures. If there is agreement, then criterion-related validity is established. If the two data

CONCLUSION

Surveys offer an effective way of collecting quantitative research data from large groups or populations, which can readily be analysed. There are a variety of survey methods within the approach and the skill is in identifying which method will best suit the topic under investigation. Survey methods offer a useful way of auditing clinical practice as well as obtaining new research data. They cannot identify causal relationships between variables or provide deeper understanding of a concept for individuals, but they can identify associations and relationships that may be open to further study. Therefore, surveys can lead on to experimental research, or qualitative studies. Survey research thus plays an important role within health care, and specifically midwifery practice.

sources are collected at about the same time, then **concurrent validity** is established. The term **predictive validity** is used in relation to how well the data collected can be used to predict something that will happen in the future. Predictive validity will be established if data collected at a later date by other means confirm the findings of the earlier survey.

Construct validity is an indication of how well the construct under study is assessed. It is usually related to concepts such as stress, anxiety, pain and social support, each of which can be difficult to define and measure.

CHAPTER SUMMARY

This chapter has highlighted that:

Surveys are quantitative and nonexperimental, the main purpose of which is to collect data about prevalence, distribution and inter-relationships of variables.

The stages of a survey are usually:

◆ Establish the research question

◆ Undertake the literature review

◆ Select the design and plan the study

◆ Pilot the design and finalize the plan

◆ Collect the data

◆ Perform the analysis

◆ Write the report and publish

The most used survey method is the questionnaire. Consider:

◆ The types of question used – open or closed

◆ The types of scale used – Likert, semantic differential, visual analogue, Guttman

◆ Distribution and return of questionnaire.

Other survey methods include interviews: face-to-face, telephone.

The Delphi survey is for obtaining judgements or consensus from a panel of experts.

The quality of the survey is dependent on:

◆ a good design

◆ high degree of reliability and validity.

Audits may use the same methods of data collection and analysis as surveys and this may be a midwife's first introduction to data handling.

REFERENCES

Bell J 1987 Doing your research project: a guide for first-time researchers in education and social science. Open University Press, Milton Keynes

Bick D E, MacArthur C 1995 Attendance, content and relevance of the six week postnatal examination. Midwifery 11(2): 69–73

Blaxter L, Hughes C, Tight M 1996 How to research. Open University Press, Buckingham

Bond S, Bond J 1982 A Delphi survey of clinical nursing research priorities. Journal of Advanced Nursing 7: 565–575

Butterworth T 1995 Identifying the characteristics of optimum practice: findings from a survey of practice experts in nursing, midwifery and health visiting. Journal of Advanced Nursing 22(1): 24–32

Cline M, Herman J, Shaw E, Morton RD 1992 Standardisation of the visual analogue scale. Nursing Research 41(6): 378–380

Crosby F, Ventura M R, Feldman M J 1989 Examination of a survey methodology: Dillman's Total Design Method. Nursing Research 38(1): 57–58

Czaja R, Blair J 1996 Designing surveys: a guide to decisions and procedures. Pine Forge Press, London

Dillman D 1978 Mail and telephone surveys: the Total Design Method. John Wiley, New York

Everett A 1993 Piercing the veil of the future: a review of the Delphi method of research. Professional Nurse Dec: 181–162

Fink A, Kosecoff J 1985 How to conduct surveys. CA Sage Publications, Newbury Park, CA

Garcia J, Redshaw M, Fitzsimons B, Keene J 1998 First class delivery: a national survey of women's views of maternity care. Audit Commission, London

Gift AG 1989 Visual analogue scales: measurement of subjective phenomena. Nursing Research 38(5): 286–288

Goodman C M 1987 The Delphi technique: a critique. Journal of Advanced Nursing 12: 729–734

Hicks C 1995 A factor analytic study of midwives' attitudes to research. Midwifery 11(1): 11–17

Holroyd E, Yin-King L, Wong Pu-yuk L, You Kwok-hong F, Leung Shuk-lin B 1997 Hong Kong Chinese women's perception of support from midwives during labour. Midwifery 13(2): 66–72

Howe T 1995 Measurement scales in health care settings. Nurse Researcher 2(4): 30–37

Jowett S, Shanley E 1993 Approaches to analysis and interpretation. Nurse Researcher 1(2): 44–51

Lee K A, Kieckhefer G M 1989 Measuring human responses using visual analogue scales. Western Journal of Nursing Research 11: 128–132

Linstone H A, Turoff M 1975 The Delphi survey. Method, techniques and applications. Addison-Wesley, Menlo Park, CA

McColl E 1993 Questionnaire design and construction. Nurse Researcher 1(2): 16–25

McKenna H P 1994 The Delphi technique: a worthwhile research approach for nursing? Journal of Advanced Nursing 19(6): 1221–1225

Mason V 1989 Women's experience of maternity care – a survey manual. HMSO, London

Meldrum P, Purton P, Maclennan B B, Twaddle S 1994 Moving toward a common understanding in maternity services. Midwifery 10(3): 165–170

Miller D C 1991 Handbook of research design and social measurement, 5th edn. Sage Publications, London

Mitchell M, Jolley J 1996 Research design explained, 3rd edn. Harcourt Brace, London

Moser C A, Kalton G 1971 Survey methods in social investigation, 2nd edn. Heinemann, London

Newell R 1994 The structured interview. Nurse Researcher 1(3): 14–22

Norusis M J 1990 The SPSS guide to data analysis, release 4. SPSS, Chicago, IL

Oppenheim A N 1992 Questionnaire design, interviewing and attitude measurement, 2nd edn. Pinter, London

Parahoo K 1997 Nursing research: principles, process and issues. Macmillan, Basingstoke

Polit D F, Hungler B P 1995 Nursing research: principles and methods, 5th edn. JB Lippincott, London

Priest J, McColl E, Thomas L, Bond S 1995 Developing and refining a new measurement tool. Nurse Researcher 2(4): 69–81

Procter S, Hunt M 1994 Using the Delphi survey technique to develop a professional definition of nursing for analysing nursing workload. Journal of Advanced Nursing 19(4): 1003–1014

Proud J, Murphy-Black T 1997 Choice of scan: how much info do women receive before ultrasound? British Journal of Midwifery 5(3): 144–147

Robinson J 1996 It's only a questionnaire: ethics in social science research. British Journal of Midwifery 4(1): 41–44

Robinson S, Owen H 1994 Retention in midwifery: findings from a longitudinal study of midwives' careers. In: Robinson S, Thompson A M (ed) Midwives' research and childbirth, vol 3. Chapman & Hall, London, ch 8, p 175–232

Smith H W 1975 Strategies of social research. The methodological imagination. Prentice Hall, London

Strachan H 1996 The future direction of nursing informatics in the UK: a Delphi study. Information Technology in Nursing 8(3): 11–14

Sudman S 1976 Applied sampling. Academic Press, New York

Sudman S, Bradburn M 1982 Asking questions: a practical guide to questionnaire design. Jossey-Bass, San Francisco, CA

Treece E W, Treece J W 1986 Elements of research in nursing. CV Mosby, St Louis, MO

Wagstaff P J 1998 Research in the clinical area: the ethical issues. Nursing Standard 12(28): 33–36

Wessex Institute 1997 Wessex Confidential Enquiry into Stillbirths and Deaths in Infancy (CESDI): incorporating Wessex Perinatal and Infant Mortality Surveys. Wessex Institute for Health Research and Development – incorporating Public Health Medicine, annual report for 1996. University of Southampton, Southampton

Williamson S, Thomson A M 1996 Women's satisfaction with antenatal care in a changing maternity service. Midwifery 12(4): 198–204

5

An introduction to statistics in midwifery research

Elizabeth Cluett

INTRODUCTION

The Department of Health document *Changing Childbirth* (Department of

Health 1993, p. 5) unequivocally states that 'every woman has unique needs' and 'maternity care must be woman centred'. This philosophy underpins the practice of most midwives and many patterns of maternity care provision (Flint et al 1989, Bryar 1991, Wraight et al 1993, Hundley et al 1994). This unique and individual approach appears to conflict with **statistics**, which is about aggregating events numerically and using them to describe and predict to general populations. Yet it is the great variability that exists between individuals that makes statistical analyses essential in evaluating many forms of health care.

If practitioners were to extrapolate from the experience of one woman (or group of women) to another woman or group, the uniqueness of the women would most probably result in inappropriate care being offered to the second woman. Statistical processes are able to help quantify that variability, to help practitioners identify how much variability is due to the natural uniqueness of individuals, how much due to chance and how much due to the treatments under consideration. This information can then be used to form the basis of individual management and care and the decision-making processes between the woman and her carers to provide what is best for her. Reid (1993) suggests that there is an art of statistics, which is appreciating what statistics can and cannot offer. Mastery in the art of statistics enables midwives to offer every woman high-quality, woman-centred care. So midwives must be able to understand the basics of statistics to enable them to evaluate research designs, interpret findings effectively and communicate the conclusions to the women they care for.

The use of statistics is not restricted to research but is an integral part of midwifery practice. The data we record at every delivery contributes to subsequent planning of services related to the health, education and social structure of our society. The confidential enquiries into maternal deaths and more recently perinatal deaths use statistics as well as individual cases to influence clinical practice. Statistical evidence can support midwifery practice through clinical audit and quality assurance, which can facilitate the appropriate resourcing of services.

This chapter aims to provide an introduction to statistics that will enable the midwife to understand the key principles, terms and findings that they will encounter in reading and evaluating research reports. It is not intended to enable midwives to undertake statistical analysis within a research project. Statistical analysis is the domain of statisticians, and when undertaking research midwives should always seek appropriate statistical support to ensure high-quality research design and analysis.

ETHICS AND STATISTICS

Statistics can neither be ethical nor unethical, but Altman (1982) highlights the fact that misuse of statistics is unethical. Just as it is unethical to falsify documents, unintentionally or not, so it is equally unethical to present incorrect statistics or use statistical tests inappropriately. One way of considering the correct and therefore ethical use of statistics is to establish whether statistical advice was sought in its compilation and whether the statistical component was reviewed prior to publication.

There is a generally held belief that statistics can be made to say anything you want – hence their popularity with politicians. Here again, the midwife can assess the ethical use of statistics. Once data has been obtained there is a temptation to look for links and test for them, even though these associations have not been planned into the method. The danger is that the unplanned analysis could result in relationships being detected between variables where there is a potential for bias across the groups for that variable. For example, suppose a study set up to consider the impact of continuity of carer on length of labour then analyses the impact of antenatal preparation on overall labour length. Subdividing the original study group by antenatal preparation may result in uneven secondary groups. More importantly, individual characteristics that would affect the relationship between education and length of labour may have been screened out to meet the criteria of the prime study on continuity of carer. So there should be evidence that the statistical analysis was planned along with the method. This would suggest that suitable attempts have been taken to ensure valid use of statistical methods.

It is unethical to undertake research on clients using a sample size too small to provide useful information or so large that clients are studied needlessly. Midwives could not be expected to calculate these **power calculations** but, when reading any paper, check whether appropriate calculations were done prior to the undertaking of the study.

Statistics cannot be evaluated separately from the research design, as they can only be as good as the study to which they are related. Thus it is important to evaluate all aspects of the research design, including the validity and reliability of the study, representativeness of the sample to the population, the inclusion criteria and the many other facets of a good research design.

PRESENTATION OF STATISTICS

The way statistics are presented can either encourage or dissuade you from deeper consideration. This is regrettable and the advice must be to remember that presentation is just a shop window; to assess the quality of the goods you do need to explore further. This means reading the tables, graphs and statistics and considering the information they are presenting to you. Tables can condense information. A range of descriptive data about a client group can be enclosed in one small table instead of a long paragraph. This saves you time reading and makes comparisons across the groups easier. It is also quicker to refer back to a table to check a point rather than trying to find a detail in a text paragraph. Graphs can give a clear picture of the pattern of an event and hence are considered helpful when describing and/or exploring available information (Gore 1982a, Matthews et al 1990). This is useful to remember if you ever need to present numerical information yourself. Scatter graphs are particularly useful for showing the relationship between one variable and another. For example, a scatter graph was used to illustrate the relationship between the body mass index of postnatal mothers and measurement variability of midwives undertaking the symphysis–fundal distance (Cluett et al 1995). All graphs should have a concise and precise title and both the axes must be labelled, the x axis being horizontal and the y axis being vertical. There should be a key for any symbols used. Look carefully at the information around the graph/chart, as the use of breaks in the scales or a logarithmic scale to transform data, which are legitimate processes, can affect the first impressions given by the graph. It should be possible to understand the graph without reference to the text. Where there is more than one graph on the same type of data, the scales and keys should be consistent, to aid comparisons. Frequency graphs are where the x axis is the characteristic being considered and the y axis indicates the number of times each characteristic occurred. This kind of graph enables you to visualize the distribution pattern of the data.

Data management includes the way data is prepared for analysis. Care must be taken to ensure that data is correctly entered into the computer package. Therefore it is advisable that the accuracy of data entry is checked. In addition, statistical packages need to be operated correctly, so while it may be possible to undertake data entry and analysis in a computer yourself it may be appropriate to have it checked either by a colleague or professionally, as human errors linked to computer use are on the increase (Roberts et al 1997). Incomplete data should be identified and cannot be part of the analysis, but lost data should be accounted for in the results. If statistical packages are used for analysis then it is advisable to identify in the results which package was used and reference it, as different packages can give slightly different results.

TYPES OF STATISTICS

There are two main types of statistics, **descriptive** and **inferential**. Descriptive statistics involve the use of numbers to paint a picture of the information. Descriptive statistics are part of everyday midwifery practice, such as the Korner data on admissions and workloads, the percentages of normal births, caesarean sections or breastfeeding rates within a maternity unit. Maternity statistics released by the Department of Health (1997) are a good example of descriptive statistics. The main descriptive statistics are those relating to measures of **central tendency** or averages and those related to **measures of dispersal** or spread.

Inferential statistics enable some inference to be made about the relationship between the variables, which may be **causal** or **correlational**. They are used to indicate what might happen in the same circumstances to a larger or similar group of people, or to move from the sample to the population from which that sample is drawn. So inferential statistics can help practitioners predict what might be happening in general, or what might happen in the future. Associated with this prediction is an evaluation of the strength of that prediction, i.e. how much reliance you can place on the inference.

Number groups or levels of measurement

Before considering specific statistics it is important to understand the way data is classified, sometimes called levels of measurement (Table 5.1). Statistical tests are selected depending on the classification of the data involved – hence the importance of understanding these groupings before considering other statistical processes.

Table 5.1 Summary of the characteristics for the levels of data

| Criteria | Categorical | | Numerical | |
	Nominal	Ordinal	Interval	Ratio
Equivalence	Yes	Yes	Yes	Yes
In progressive order	No	Yes	Yes	Yes
Identical distances between values	No	No	Yes	Yes
'Zero' is present	No	No	No	Yes

There are two main levels, **categorical** and **numerical**. Categorical can be subdivided into **nominal** and **ordinal**. Nominal data is where numbers are used to classify items instead of a title or name. Data expressed in either/or formats come into this classification, for example Yes/No responses or Male/Female. There may be more than two groups, as for marital status – married, single, widowed and divorced. Often a number is used to identify the group, but if you can replace the number with a name then the data is categorical. For example, the number 11 bus takes me to work; it could be called the hospital bus, it would still be the same route. Nominal data shows equivalence only. So you cannot add two number 11 buses together to reach the university, which is on the 22 bus route. For this type of data the only information that can be given is the frequency, i.e. the number of items in each group, and percentages.

Ordinal data is where the items are in rank order, for example pain scores in labour from 0, no pain to 10, excruciating pain. Here the numbers show equivalence and relative progression, so 4 always indicates more pain than 2, but two 2s may not equal 4. Thus the distance or interval between each number may not be the same. As with nominal data, there are considerable limitations on the mathematical functions that can be performed on this type of data.

Numerical data is also divided into subgroups, **interval** and **ratio**. Interval data has numbers in rank order with the same distance between each of the numbers. There is, however, no absolute zero, i.e. zero is allocated arbitrarily. For example –5°C is a valid temperature, whereas –5 babies is nonsense. There are very few examples of interval data, calendar and temperature scales being the best known, and although interval data is included here for completeness, the majority of numerical data will be ratio data. Ratio data has the same features as interval data but additionally there is an absolute zero. Therefore a 10% increase always results in the same amount of change, hence the name ratio data. Ratio data is the most powerful type of data and all mathematical processes can be performed on this data. Characteristics such as age, birthweight, length of labour and many others are examples of ratio data.

Numerical data can also be subdivided into **discrete data** and **continuous data** where discrete data is anything that only occurs in whole numbers, such as babies: you cannot have 0.5 of a baby. Continuous numbers are where every decimal division between each of the whole numbers is possible, such as 0.25 litres of blood.

When deciding which sort of data is involved it is important to consider what the numbers are representing. A good example of this is the Apgar score. The score for each characteristic is 0, 1 or 2. At first glance this appears numerical in nature, but consider heart rate: a score of 0 is given if there is no heart beat, 1 if the rate is under 100 and 2 if it is above 100. The distances between these stages are clearly not the same, although there is a progressive improvement, and thus this data is categorical, specifically ordinal in nature.

Descriptive statistics

Measures of central tendency – averages

There are three forms of average. The first and most widely used is the **mean**, sometimes called the arithmetic mean. This is obtained by adding the score of all the measurements together and dividing by the number of measurements (Box 5.1).

Box 5.1 The formula for calculating a mean

The formula is: $\dfrac{\Sigma x}{n} = \bar{x}$

where the individual measurement is x,

the bar over the x, $\bar{x}$, is the symbol for the mean,

the symbol Σ (a Greek capital sigma) means the sum of, and the letter n is used to represent the number of measurements obtained.

These symbols are often used within articles and it is therefore useful to be able to recognize them.

The mean may not be one of the original measurements, or even a whole number, and may not usefully represent the original information. For example, a batch of uniforms made to a mean size may not fit any of the midwives! So the mean is most useful when dealing with data that is numerical and continuous, such as length of labour; it is sensible to talk about 1.5 hours of labour but not 1.5 babies. It can be used with categorical data; for example, the mean pain score between women using different forms of analgesia might be a useful indicator of labour pain experienced. However the limitation, the variable nature of amount of difference between any two values, i.e. 3 and 4 compared to 4 and 5 should be identified. The mean is considered the preferable measure of central tendency when the data is symmetrically distributed.

The **median** is the midpoint when all measurements are in numerical order, so there are as many numbers or measurements above it as there are below it. This could be called the halfway observation or the 50% point. This value may be one of the original items or, where there is an even number of items in the group it may be a value midway between two measurements. The median is most commonly used where the data is not continuous, or where the distribution is not symmetrical. Growth patterns, such as infant height and weight, or antenatal fundal height assessment usually use the median. As both the mean and the median give useful information about the data it may be appropriate that both are given.

The **mode**, which indicates the most popular value in any group of values, or the one that occurs most frequently, is the third and least used measure of central tendency. This may have no relationship to the central point of the group or the mean, but is always one of the original items. There may be two or more values that occur with equal frequency; when shown as a block graph (also called a bar chart) this shows two separate high points.

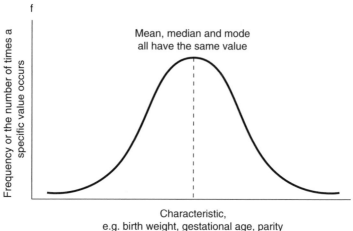

Figure 5.1 A normal distribution curve

Normal distribution

The normal curve was first calculated mathematically by a man called Karl Friedrich Gauss in 1795; hence it is sometimes know as the gaussian curve. Figure 5.1 shows a normal distribution curve. It has three specific features:

◆ it is symmetrical around one central point
◆ the mean, median and mode all occur at the same point at the centre of the curve
◆ the values that define the curve are continuous and extend at each extreme to infinity.

As a result of these characteristics the area underneath the curve can always be subdivided into regions that represent a fixed percentage of the population under study. This remains true regardless of how the group's values are clustered around the central point. The presence of data that are normally distributed is of special importance in statistics, as many of the methods of analysis and statistical tests are chosen depending on whether or not the data available demonstrate a normal distribution. When the mean, median and mode of a data set have different values the distribution is skewed. The curve may be skewed to the left or right, as shown in Figure 5.2.

Measure of dispersal

The range

A measure of dispersal refers to the spread of the data around the mean (or median). The **range** is the most common way of doing this, the range being

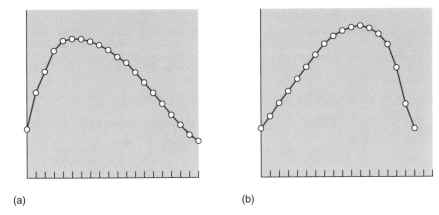

(a)   (b)

Figure 5.2 Graphs to show distribution that is skewed to the left (**a**) or the right (**b**)

the minimum and maximum values of the data. The limitation of the range is that knowing the most extreme values need not indicate the pattern of the data. The values could be mainly at the centre with one or two extremes, or evenly distributed throughout. For this reason a better way of describing the spread or dispersal is through the **standard deviation**.

The standard deviation

The standard deviation (SD) indicates the degree or amount of variability within any group of scores in relation to the mean score. The SD indicates the average distance individual scores are away from the mean score of the group, which can be in a positive or a negative direction. The larger the SD the more spread out the individual scores are, i.e. the further the majority of individual scores are away from the mean. A small SD shows that the majority of individual scores are close to the mean. An SD of 0 means that every individual score is the same, as there is no variability. Most textbooks covering statistics give a step-by-step guide to calculating the standard deviation but I would recommend Clegg (1982) as being particularly clear to anyone undertaking this for the first time. An example to illustrate how the SD can provide an insight into a group is given in Box 5.2.

These two groups of mothers could be quite different, despite having the same mean and range. This may be clinically important information: group 1 may be multiparae with and without complications in labour; group 2 may be nulliparae.

The standard deviation has a unique relationship with the normal distribution curve, as the area under the normal curve can always be divided into areas defined by the SD. One standard deviation from the mean will

Box 5.2 An example for standard deviation

Comparison of length of labour for two groups of 12 women:

Group 1	Group 2
2, 2, 3, 3, 3, 4, 4, 5, 5, 5, 24, 24	2, 5, 5, 5, 5, 6, 6, 6, 6, 7, 7, 24
The range is 2–24 hours	The range is 2–24 hours
The mean is 7	The mean is 7
The standard deviation (SD) is 7.6	The standard deviation (SD) is 5.2

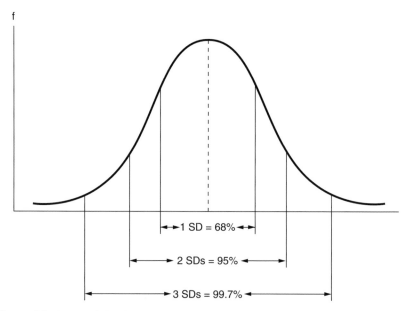

Figure 5.3 A normal distribution curve showing the areas under the curve, and their percentages, described by the standard deviation

always define the same percentage of the area under the curve, 34% (some texts calculate this to a greater number of decimal places but 34% is precise enough for the majority of situations). Consideration of an area under the curve of one SD above and below the mean indicates that 68% of the individual scores for the group lie within that region.

Figure 5.3 shows the relationship between the normal distribution curve and the SD, including how the sum of two SDs on either side of the mean incorporates 95% of the individual scores of the group. This is used in defining normal ranges, which is described as the mean plus or minus 2 SD, written ±2 SD. The sum of three SDs includes 99.7% of the group. Regardless

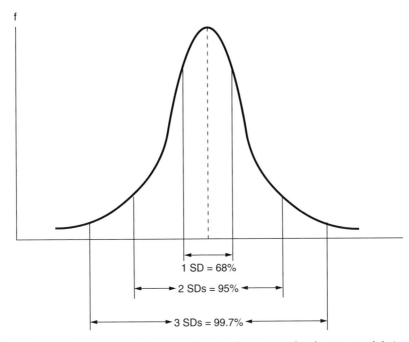

Figure 5.4 A normal distribution curve showing the areas under the curve and their percentages when the standard deviation is small

of the size of the standard deviation, these percentages remain true. A tall and thin curve occurs when the SD is small (Fig. 5.4) and a short, broad curve occurs when the SD is large (Fig. 5.5). An image of the distribution of the data can be achieved by knowing the mean of any group and its SD.

Variance

Another measure of dispersal is **variance**. It is obtained as one of the steps in the calculation of the standard deviation and, like the SD, is used when the mean of the data is the appropriate average. The variance is the standard deviation squared. As with SD, the larger the variance the greater the spread or distribution of the scores within the group. The variance is used in a series of statistical tests called analysis of variance or ANOVA, which will be mentioned later in this chapter.

Standard error

The **standard error** (SE) can sometimes be confused with standard deviation. As described above, the standard deviation is about the variability of individual

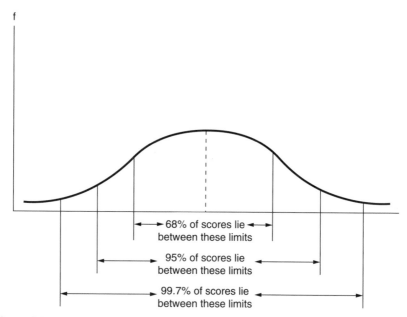

f

68% of scores lie
between these limits

95% of scores lie
between these limits

99.7% of scores lie
between these limits

Figure 5.5 A normal distribution curve showing the areas under the curve and their percentages when the standard deviation is large

scores around the mean of that group. If every score for a whole population was collected we could be certain that the mean was correct. In reality, we are usually only able to access a sample from the population. Different samples from the same population would give different means. For example, the mean length of labour for a group of 100 women might be 8.5 hours, while that for a different group of 100 women might be 7.9 hours and for a third group of women 9.1 hours. Thus the mean of any one sample is likely to vary slightly from the mean of the total population from which that sample is drawn.

If it were possible to obtain the mean length of labour from many samples, a graph could be drawn of the mean values obtained. This graph would show that the means from repeated samples form a normal distribution curve. Therefore it is possible to calculate the standard deviation of the mean, which is the standard error (SE), hence the potential for confusion. So while the SD always reflects the variability of individual scores in a group and will be of the same magnitude regardless of how large the sample is, the mean of the sample will get closer to the population mean as the size of the sample increases. Thus the SE will get progressively smaller as the sample size increases. So the SE can be considered as an indicator of how much reliance can be placed on the sample mean as a reflection of the population mean. In reality, it is not possible to keep undertaking the same study to obtain lots of mean values for each sample, so there is a formula that allows the SE to be calculated from one sample. Polit and Hungler (1997) and Swinscow (1996) provide a good explanation of standard error. Although I have discussed SE here because of its similarity to the SD, standard error is often considered along with inferential statistics because of its association with samples and their relationship to a population.

Centiles and the interquartile range

When the median is the average, centiles are used to describe the dispersal of the data. Centiles are imaginary lines that divide the data into regions, where each region covers a known percentage of the data. Having calculated the median, which is the 50% line, the next centiles usually calculated are the 25% and 75% lines, dividing the data into four. The measure of dispersal for the data is the distance between the 25% and 75% (also called 25th and 75th) centiles; this is the **interquartile range** (IQR). Rowntree (1981, p. 52) calls this a 'mini range'. If the interquartile range is small then half the group have scores that lie close to the median. If the interquartile range is large the variability of individual scores will be greater and further from the median. The interquartile range is not influenced by individual scores at the extremes of the data and is therefore considered to provide a representative picture of score dispersal. Johnson et al (1997) used the median and IQR to compare the time intervals to amniotomy in their study of early or selective amniotomy. Other centiles, in pairs, are used, the most common being the 10th and 90th centile and the 3rd and 97th centile. Measurements between the 10th and 90th centile are usually considered normal, while readings outside these centiles are indicative of potential complications.

Probability, p values and significance

Probability and the 'p' value

An understanding of **probability** is required for inferential statistics. Probability is an assessment of the chances that a specific event might occur between two or more possible outcomes. For example, the probability that the next baby will be male is 1 out of 2. One definition could be:

> Probability is the likelihood that an event might happen, compared to the total number of times it is possible for that event to occur.

This type of probability is called model probability (Campbell and Machin 1993), as the number of possibilities is clear, so any one birth must be one of those possibilities. This type of probability is used in genetic counselling, where the model is the inheritance patterns for various conditions. Frequency probability is when the estimate of the likelihood of an event happening is based on previous experience, or the frequency with which the event has happened in previous samples. For example, the probability of receiving an epidural in the local maternity unit is 20%, this figure being calculated by assessing how many women received an epidural in the preceding months. Frequency probability is the most often used in research. The third type of probability is subjective probability, which is when the probability is based on a reasonable belief rather than empirical data; for example, the probability of day trips to the moon in the next century is low, or is it? Campbell and Machin (1993) give a good explanation of the main types of probability, with examples.

Inferential statistics rely on the assessment of probability to consider if one set of women is the same as the next and if a new care option would work in the wider pregnant population because it helped one group. It does this by answering the question: Could the outcome of the new treatment/management be due to chance and not the research actions? Hicks (1996) refers to this chance element as the 'random error factor'. This negative approach is because it is always easier to disprove something than to prove it. The **null hypothesis** is consistent with this negative approach. As explained in Chapter 3, the null hypothesis states there is *no* difference between the study groups. The hope is that research findings will disprove or reject the null hypothesis, indicating a difference between groups. So, usually, research studies are looking for a small probability that the result was due to chance; and hence by implication the result was due to the new treatment.

Probability can be expressed as a percentage, or in a ratio; thus a 50:50 chance is a 50% chance or an equal chance, while a 1 in 5 chance could be expressed as 20% or 5:1. Probability is given the symbol p (some texts use an upper case P) and is usually expressed as a decimal number between 0 and 1. A value of 1 means that the event is an absolute certainty: every person born will eventually die. Zero indicates an absolute impossibility. Linking the negative approach of statistics and Hicks's (1996) random error factor means that the p value could be interpreted as indicating the likelihood that the research findings are due to random errors, which are unpredictable or occur by chance. Clegg (1982) provides a clear description of the nature of probability for those who have not dealt with this concept before.

Probability is quantified to enable researchers and practitioners to understand how much reliance they can place on the information available, usually research findings from experimental studies or correlational surveys. The smaller the p value the less likely it is that the results obtained were due to chance. Table 5.2 lists some p values and how they can be interpreted.

With any probability calculation there is always the possibility of error. So

Table 5.2 A list of the most commonly seen p values, with their interpretations

p value	No. of times 'it'* would occur by chance	No. of times 'it' would be due to the 'care'	Significant/ not significant
$p = 0.5$	5 times out of 10	5 times out of 10	Not significant
$p = 0.3$	3 times out of 10	7 times out of 10	Not significant
$p = 0.1$	1 time in 10	9 times out of 10	Not significant
$p = 0.05$	5 times out of 100	95 times out of 100	Significant
$p = 0.02$	2 times out of 100	98 times out of 100	Significant
$p = 0.01$	1 time in 100	99 times out of 100	Significant
$p = 0.005$	5 times out of 1000	995 times out of 1000	Significant
$p = 0.001$	1 time in 1000	999 times out of 1000	Significant
$p = 0.0001$	1 time in 10 000	9999 times out of 10 000	Significant

* 'it' represents the outcome measure; for example, 'it' could be the improvement in maternal satisfaction due to support in labour.

even when the probability is very small, say $p = 0.05$, suggesting that the outcome was due to the treatment, there still remains that small possibility that the outcome was due to chance. Equally, if the probability is large, say $p = 0.2$, which suggests that the outcome was due to chance, there is still the possibility that the obtained result was due to the new treatment. These two situations are well recognized and are called **type I and type II errors**. These errors are always considered in relation to the null hypothesis.

◆ A type I error is when a null hypothesis that is true is rejected.
◆ A type II error is when a null hypothesis that is false is accepted.

Level of significance

In clinical research the main fear is of concluding that a new treatment is of benefit when it is not, i.e. rejecting the null hypothesis incorrectly or making a type 1 error. To reduce the chances of a type 1 error, null hypotheses are only rejected when the probability that the findings were due to chance is very small, i.e. the p value is small. The level of significance is the p value at which the researchers deem the chances of getting a type 1 error to be small enough for the purposes of their study. In most studies, $p = 0.05$ is accepted as the level of significance, i.e. when there is a 5% chance of the result being due to chance. So where $p = 0.05$ or less the results are said to be **significant** and where $p = 0.05$ or more the results are **not significant** (Table 5.2). However, on occasions, for example if there are known side-effects of the new treatment, researchers may decide they want the chance of a type 1 error to be even smaller. Then $p=0.01$ is adopted, which means that there is only a 1% chance of the results being due to chance.

Statistical significance must NOT be confused with clinical significance. It is possible for a study to show a statistically significant difference between the study groups but for that difference to have no clinical significance at all. For example, research comparing current care to a 'new' management of the first stage of labour may reduce the length of labour by 10 minutes. The statistical analysis might indicate that the difference between the groups is significant, i.e. unlikely to be due to chance, but midwives know that a difference of 10 minutes has no real clinical significance. Thus the meaning of the word 'significant' is fundamentally different in the two contexts. So while statistics may be useful in indicating where there is a difference or not, only practitioners can decide whether the difference is important to their practice.

Inferential statistics

Tests of significance

Inferential statistics enable some inference to be made about the relationship between variables. The tests to achieve this are sometimes known as tests of significance because they assist practitioners in evaluating whether there is a significant difference between subject groups in experimental and correlational studies. This significance is expressed as a precise mathematical value and indicates how much reliability can be attributed to the difference found between groups; in other words, could the findings be due to chance or is it reasonable to attribute the findings to the independent variable under review?

Tests of significance can be subdivided into **parametric** and **nonparametric** tests. Parametric tests are considered to be the more powerful group of tests or the more sensitive tests, because the following criteria must be met:

◆ the dependent variable must be a continuous measurement, i.e. numerical data at either interval or ratio level
◆ the dependent variable should fit a normal distribution curve across the study population or be able to be transformed into a normal distribution by use of logarithms
◆ the standard deviations from the groups being studied must be of approximately the same magnitude.

Nonparametric tests only require the data to be of nominal or ordinal level and can be used if there is doubt as to whether the data fits a normal distribution. While it is possible to use nonparametric tests instead of parametric tests, this is not done as they are less sensitive. This would result in wider margins of error and less reliance could be placed on the research outcomes, so the null hypothesis might be accepted, suggesting that there was no difference between the groups, when in fact a difference did exist. In addition, nonparametric tests are unsuitable for more complex analysis, such as where several factors are being considered at the same time. Thus wherever possible parametric tests should be used.

If a causal relationship is being investigated the null hypothesis can be rejected or supported by evaluating whether there is a difference between the means of two or more groups for the facet under consideration. The aim is to elucidate whether there is a difference between the means and whether it could have occurred by chance or not. These tests can be used to evaluate whether there is any difference between the groups in terms of characteristics such as age, weight or any other feature common to both groups. This is useful for surveys where the aim is to compare descriptive characteristics across groups of people. The null hypothesis in these situations is not usually stated but would be:

> there is no difference in age, weight, ethnic origin, and so on, across the study groups.

In well-organized randomized control trials, tests for such differences should show no difference between the groups, as the process of randomization should have equalized this type of variable across the groups. When tests for the difference between means are used to compare the mean scores for the dependent variable across the groups in a randomized control trial, then the aim is to consider causality. The null hypothesis would now be expressed as no difference in the dependent variable (outcome) regardless of whether participants received the independent variable (experimental treatment) or not. For example, in the study comparing one-to-one care, could the difference in analgesic between the experimental and control groups be due to the one-to-one care or to chance (Hofmeyr et al 1991)?

Correlation and its associated tests are considered in more detail later in the chapter, but parametric or nonparametric and difference in means or correlation tests can be combined:

◆ parametric and difference in means
◆ parametric and correlational
◆ nonparametric and difference in means
◆ nonparametric and correlational.

This chapter cannot include all the possible tests, so a few of the more frequently used tests are considered. For further information on statistical tests you would be advised to refer to a statistics text (see further reading list) or a statistician.

Parametric tests for differences between means

The *t* tests

The original *t* test was devised by William Gosset, who was prevented from publishing under his own name and instead called himself 'Student'; hence it is often referred to as Student's *t* test. There are two main types of *t* test, the independent *t* test and the dependent *t* test.

The independent t test

This tests the null hypothesis by considering whether the mean scores for both groups are similar or not; in other words, could the two groups have been drawn from the same population? For example, is the mean length of labour for women in water so similar to that for women on a bed that they might all have had the same care? Remember, to use this test the data must be continuous, of interval or ratio level and approximately normally distributed, which can be checked by plotting the data on a graph prior to analysis.

The groups should show a degree of homogeneity with respect to the variable under consideration. This implies that the variables are of approximately the same numerical magnitude, so one group cannot have scores in the hundreds while the other is in single numbers. For example, the *t* tests could not compare maternal weights in pregnancy with neonatal birth weights, but it could compare the birthweight of a mother with that of her infant.

It is possible to compare a group of 50 with one of 60, as groups do not have to be of the same size for the independent *t* test. *T* tests can be undertaken when sample sizes are small, about 10 in each group; however, the smaller the sample the greater the difference will have to be in the outcomes measured in the groups before the test identifies any significant difference.

To calculate the *t* test you need to know the number of scores, the mean and the SDs for each group. The *t* test is then calculated using a formula and calculator, or a computer statistics programme. This gives you a number, which is looked up in a *t*-test statistical table to find the appropriate *p* value. Such tables are found in the back of most statistical texts. However, statistical computer packages such as SPSS (Puri 1996) are now widely available and do this automatically. Waldenstrom et al (1997) used *t* tests to compare baseline data such as maternal age at delivery and parity in a study comparing care provided in a birth centre with standard hospital care. Here the *t* test was used to check that effective randomization had occurred and that there was no difference between the groups in relation to stated demographic data. This result is what you would expect in a randomized trial.

The dependent *t* test

The dependent or paired *t* test is used when there are two sets of readings, such as before and after an intervention, from one group of subjects. There must be the same number of readings in each set. If individual readings are missing the pair is excluded from the analysis. After ensuring that the criteria for parametric tests have been met, the calculation of the paired *t* test is undertaken, following the appropriate formulae or using a computer. As before, this gives a numerical figure to which a *p* value is associated that indicates whether the null hypothesis should be supported or rejected.

One- and two-tailed tests

Several statistical tests can be subdivided into one- or two-tailed tests, including the *t* tests. A one-tailed test looks for a change in one direction versus no change between the groups. For example, a one-tailed test on infants having phototherapy would look for an improvement in serum bilirubin levels, as the anticipated direction of the change is known. Two-tailed tests look for change in either direction, i.e. an improvement or deterioration, compared to no change. For example in a study considering two different perineal suturing techniques, a two-tailed test would consider if the rate of healing was longer or shorter, or made no difference. It is important to select the correct test, otherwise there is potential for missing a difference between the groups. In practice, it is advisable to use two-tailed tests to eliminate the danger of missing a change in the opposite direction from that expected.

Nonparametric tests for differences between means

Mann–Whitney U test

The Mann–Whitney U test is used to consider the difference between two separate groups where the data are at ordinal level, i.e. in ranked order. This test is the nonparametric equivalent of the independent *t* test and can be used where the number of individual scores in each group is different. It can be used with relatively small numbers in each group, such as 10. However the most important feature of the Mann–Whitney U test is that it can be used to compare the means of groups where there is a skewed distribution. As with the tests described earlier, the calculation of this test using either a computer package or the appropriate statistical formulae and table, gives a single number, sometimes called the *U* value, and its associated *p* value. Mathews et al (1998) used the Mann–Whitney U test to compare data that was not normally distributed in a study of the use of folic acid prior to conception.

Wilcoxon test

The Wilcoxon signed rank test, usually referred to as the Wilcoxon test, is the nonparametric equivalent of the dependent t test. Scores should be in pairs, such as before and after treatment, and the test is used where the data do not follow a normal distribution curve. The number of pairs in the study needs to be known, as do the differences between each pair of scores. Then a single number, sometimes called the T value, is calculated with the corresponding p value, using a computer package or the appropriate statistical formulae and table. This identifies whether or not there is a significant difference. In a case-controlled study comparing nutritional differences in women paired for whether they had a normal infant or an infant with a neural tube defect, Wright (1995) used the Wilcoxon test to consider whether there were any differences in dietary elements between pairs of women. Some significant differences were identified.

The chi-squared test

The chi-squared test, the symbol for which is x^2, is well known and, although classified as a nonparametric test it can be considered separately. The test is sometimes referred to as the 'goodness of fit test' (Clegg 1982), as it considers whether the distribution pattern or frequency of the variable under consideration in one group is the same as, or 'fits', the distribution pattern in the second group. The groups and/or subgroups are considered as cells or bands and are usually presented as a contingency table. While previous tests discussed looked for differences between groups, the chi-squared test considers whether the distribution of variables across two or more cells is what was expected (Box 5.3).

There are two versions of the chi-squared test, the simple x^2, which is used when there are two groups or sets of data at nominal level, and the complex x^2, which is when there are three or more sets of data. Calculating the x^2 gives a number. You then need to consider the number of degrees of freedom for the study. The concept of degrees of freedom (df) is derived from statistical theory. While explaining the concept in detail is beyond the scope of this book, it is basically an indicator of how many readings are free to alter given the value of the other readings. It is, however, easy to calculate the df, as it is the number of scores/measurements in the data set minus the number of data sets in the study. Usually, there is one data set, so df is the number of scores minus one, written as $df = n - 1$. The chi-square value can then be looked up in significance tables for the chi-squared test for the correct level of degrees of freedom. In a study into attendance rates at the 6-week postnatal examination (Bick and MacArthur 1995), the chi-squared test was used to consider

---

Box 5.3 Example using the chi-squared test

A group of mothers are given a glass of cider; a second group are given a glass of apple juice. They are asked to score 20 neonates as cute or not. If approximately the same number of neonates are classified as cute by both groups of mothers, you could conclude that cider does not increase mothers' perceptions of 'cuteness' in babies.

Expected results:	Cider group	Apple juice group
Number of cute babies	15	15
Actual results:	Cider group	Apple juice group
Number of cute babies	19	6

In effect the chi-squared test compares what the actual result is with what the expected result would be and, if there is large difference, then the test shows that the difference is significant.

---

whether the pattern of attendance related to the pattern of marital status and parity. Their results – $x^2 = 33.53$, df = 1, $p < 0.001$ – showed a significant difference. If there was no relationship between attendance and marital status, the proportion of single women who attended would be identical to that of married women. The chi test showed that the proportions were different, so nonattenders were significantly more likely to be single.

Correlation and the associated statistical tests

Correlational research designs are when researchers explore the relationship between two series of observations. These are primarily nonexperimental designs. There may be several variables involved but there is no manipulation of variables. Retrospective design and surveys are the most common correlational studies. Correlation tests assess whether, as one variable alters, the other also changes in a predictable pattern. They do not establish a causal relationship. To illustrate the difference between causal and correlational it is useful to remember the following story. During the 1960s the birth rate increased; over the same period the number of geese rose. There was a correlation between these variables; however this does not prove that geese brought the babies.

A correlational study gives a series of results or measurements, usually in pairs. For example in a study considering maternal weight and gestation, for every weight obtained there will be corresponding data on the weeks of gestation. This can be plotted on a scatter graph as in Figure 5.6, which shows that, as pregnancy advances, maternal weight increases.

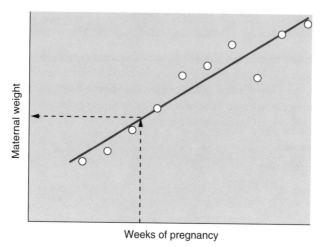

Weeks of pregnancy

Figure 5.6 A scatter graph to show a positive correlation

This is a positive correlation. The line of best fit is an imaginary line drawn through the points starting at the bottom left and moving towards the top right of the graph, indicating that, as one variable increases, the other also increases. A negative correlation is shown in Figure 5.7: as one variable increases, the other decreases. The line through the points starts in the upper left corner and travels down to the lower right corner, so as the number of days postpartum increases, the amount of lochia decreases.

In addition to knowing whether the correlation is positive or negative, the strength of the correlation should be quantified. This is indicated by a correlation coefficient, using statistical tests appropriate to the study. The correlation coefficient always lies between −1 and +1: +1 is the perfect positive correlation and −1 the perfect negative correlation. Zero indicates that there is no relationship between variables. Table 5.3 shows correlation coefficients with a possible interpretation.

The researcher and/or clinician must decide what s/he considers to be a significant correlation, depending on the nature of the variables under study. A study exploring relationship between physical measurements may require a high degree of correlation, and so a value of −8 or +8 must be identified. It is recognized that there is less likelihood of high correlations in psychological measurements such as anxiety, anger and beliefs, so lower coefficients may be anticipated. As a result, there is overlap between the categories within the table and the final interpretation is the responsibility of practitioners and is discipline- and study-dependent.

The strength of a correlation can be gauged from a graph. When the line of best fit is drawn between all the study points, the closer the individual points are to the line the stronger the correlation and the higher the coefficient will

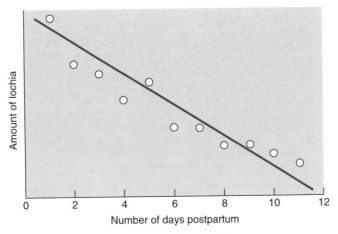

Figure 5.7 A scatter graph to show a negative correlation

Table 5.3 Correlation coefficients with a possible interpretation

Range of correlation coefficient	Interpretation
−1.0 to −0.8	A very strong to perfect negative correlation
−0.8 to −0.6	A good negative correlation
−0.6 to −0.4	A moderately negative correlation
−0.4 to −0.2	A weakly negative correlation
−0.2 to 0	A very weak negative correlation to no correlation
0 to +0.2	A very weak positive correlation to no correlation
0.2 to 0.4	A weakly positive correlation
0.4 to 0.6	A moderately positive correlation
0.6 to 0.8	A good positive correlation
0.8 to 1	A very strong to perfect positive correlation

be. Alternatively, the further the points are from the line the weaker the relationship and the lower the coefficients would be. A cluster or circle of points suggests no relationship.

Correlation coefficients

Correlation tests assume that the data is linear, and it is advisable to plot a graph to check this before calculating the coefficients. Linear relationships approximate a straight line; however, sometimes there is clearly a relationship between variables but when the scatter graph is drawn a curved relationship is noticed, as in Figures 5.8 and 5.9.

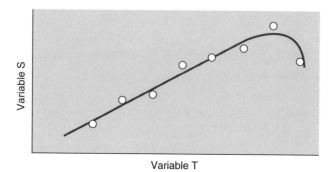

Figure 5.8 A graph illustrating a nonlinear relationship that may be due to one erroneous reading

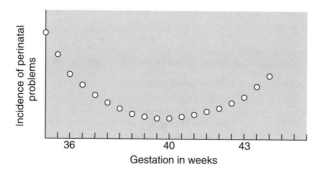

Figure 5.9 A graph illustrating a true nonlinear or curved correlation

The curve could be due to one reading, as in Figure 5.8. This may be a true reading or represent an error in the data. Ignoring the reading could be considered to be tampering with the results, while including it in any tests might lead to erroneous conclusions about the correlation. This problem is more likely to occur if the sample size is small. However outliers, or extreme values, can influence results from large studies. Where there is a true nonlinear relationship, as in Figure 5.9, advanced statistics beyond the scope of this chapter are required and you should seek statistical assistance.

Pearson's coefficient

The Pearson's coefficient or Pearson's product-moment coefficient is the most commonly used parametric correlation test. It is used when the variables are numerical. Although it is possible to calculate Pearson's coefficient manually there are many stages to the calculation and it usually requires a computer statistical package. The calculation gives a numerical value, r, between -1 and $+1$. The next step is to test for significance, to assess whether the relationship could have occurred by chance or not. This is similar to the statistics related to 'difference between the mean' tests. The test evaluates whether the r value is significantly different from zero or not. This relates to the null hypothesis, which states there is no difference. If the correlation coefficient is significantly different from zero, the null hypothesis is rejected. Obtaining the level of significance requires a further calculation, involving the size of the sample studied and the r value, and gives another numerical value, usually called t, and an associated p value. Adopting the 95% level of significance, a p value of 0.05 or less suggests a 5% or less chance of obtaining this level of correlation if there is no relationship between the two variables.

Spearman's coefficient

Spearman's coefficient is also called Spearman's rho and is a nonparametric test. It is used when evaluating the relationship between two variables where the data is ordinal or where it is uncertain whether the criteria for the parametric test, Pearson's coefficient, have been met. The data should be in ranked pairs and is best if the relationship is linear. As with Pearson's coefficient, a value between −1 and +1 is obtained. From this and the sample size an assessment of the significance can be made. Cluett et al (1995) used Spearman's rho to assess the relationship between maternal body mass index and the variability in midwives' measurements of the symphysis-pubis–fundus distance. There was a weak–moderate positive relationship, which was significant at the 95% level, or $p < 0.05$, suggesting that as body mass index increased the amount of variability in obtaining the measurements also increased.

Regression

Correlation considers the relationship between the variables obtained. Of potentially more value is the ability to predict a likely value of one variable given the other variable. This is possible if it is assumed that any change in the x axis variable, usually the independent variable, will cause a predictable change in the y axis variable, usually the dependent variable. The line of best fit can be calculated precisely and extended beyond the points actually obtained. A prediction can be made from the graph, so that the value of one variable can be predicted for any value of the other variable. In Figure 5.6 the arrowed dotted lines indicate a maternal weight estimated for a stated number of weeks into pregnancy. The 'line of best fit' was originally calculated by a scientist who concluded that if the sample was big enough there would always be a tendency for the relationship between variables to regress to the middle. This line, called the **regression line**, can be calculated using an equation based on pairs of measurements from a study sample and it describes the anticipated relationship between variables.

When more than one variable is compared with another, multiple regression analysis is undertaken. Hundley et al (1995) used multiple regression to consider which of a number of factors was most likely to predict midwives' satisfaction with the care they provided depending on whether they worked in a midwifery or consultant-led unit. They suggested that being able to make all decisions related to the provision of care in labour was the best predictor of midwives' satisfaction (Hundley et al 1995). Statistical texts provide further information on multiple regression analysis.

Other statistical terms and processes associated with inferential statistics

Confidence intervals

The **confidence interval** (CI) is a descriptive statistic indicating the population parameters for a particular characteristic. The CI indicates the magnitude of uncertainty that is associated with the mean value obtained from a sample. It gives upper and lower limits, which is a range between which the population mean is likely to lie, based on the sample's mean and standard deviation. Hicks (1996) refers to interval estimation and gives details of how to calculate the CI, with examples. The use of CIs acknowledges that research studies usually rely on information from samples but aim to project the results to the whole population, and that therefore there is the possibility of error. Assuming that the sample is representative of the population, the sample's mean and SD are likely to be different from the population's mean and SD, if only slightly. The calculation of the 95% CI enables researchers and clinicians to be confident that, if 100 independent samples were drawn from the identical population, 95% of the samples' means would lie within the range between the upper and lower confidence values. However, 5% of the samples' means might not. It is possible to calculate the CI at any percentage, but 95% is usually used as this relates to the normal distribution curve and the relationship of standard deviation to that curve. To badly misquote Aristotle and Mr Spock of *Star Trek*, the improbable is still possible, which is rather more likely than one lottery ticket winning the jackpot!

I have included CIs with inferential statistics because, although they can be used to describe population parameters, they are more commonly used in association with tests of significance. They describe the range between which the true difference between two types of management/treatment is likely to lie, based on the results of experimental research, where one group received a new treatment and the second did not. For example, a fictitious research study compared augmentation of labour with no intervention. The difference between the groups showed that the mean duration of labour was 1 hour shorter in the augmentation group, and a test of significance gave $p=0.06$, which is not statistically significant. The 95% CI was calculated to indicate the upper and lower values for the difference in length of labour – in other words, what range of differences could be expected if the same trial was repeated using different samples from the same population. In the example, a 95% CI of –0.5 to 3 hours indicates that the true impact of augmentation would most probably result in a labour that was between half-an-hour longer and 3 hours shorter compared to no intervention. So confidence intervals provide more information than a p value alone, as a p value shows the degree of support, or lack of it, that can be given to the null hypothesis whereas a CI indicates the strength of the evidence: how much impact any given management/treatment will have on the population. Confidence intervals can be presented with many other types of statistic such as numbers needed to treat (NNT) and relative risk reduction (RRR), both of which will be discussed shortly.

Confidence intervals can be calculated on most sample sizes, however the smaller the sample the wider the confidence interval and the larger the sample size the smaller the confidence interval. Gore (1982b) suggests that to halve the distance between the upper and lower confidence limits, the sample size needs to be multiplied by four.

Odds ratio

The **odds ratio** (OR) is a useful summary statistic (Campbell and Machin 1993) and can be used to report on individual studies or to summarize an overview of a topic. Its use is becoming increasingly common and therefore it is important that midwives are able to interpret information presented in this manner. An odds ratio is defined as 'the ratio of two odds' (Campbell and Machin 1993). This means that the OR compares the chances (odds) of subjects with outcome y having been in circumstances a or not with the chances of subjects not having outcome y having been in circumstances a or not.

This could be written as:

$$\frac{\text{the odds of subjects with outcome } y \text{ having been in circumstances } a \text{ or not}}{\text{the odds of subjects not having outcome } y \text{ having been in circumstances } a \text{ or not.}}$$

The number of subjects in each arm of a trial and the numbers having or not having the outcome variables under consideration are used to calculate the OR following the equation above, to give a single value that will always be greater than 0. An OR of 1.0 indicates that subjects have the same chance of having outcome *y* regardless of whether they were in circumstances *a* or not, so *a* is neither beneficial nor detrimental to *y*. An OR of less than 1 suggests that receiving the independent variable *a* is beneficial, and that subjects are less likely to get outcome *y*. An OR of greater than 1 suggests that *a* is detrimental, and that subjects are more likely to get outcome *y*. Although this is the most usual interpretation of ORs, occasionally 'benefit' and 'detriment' are reversed. Then the beneficial effect is indicated by a value greater than 1 while the detrimental effect is indicated by a value less than 1; therefore, careful reading of how the authors have interpreted their data and their presentation of results is needed.

The Cochrane Databases present odds ratios as part of the meta-analysis of most topics. They refer to the 'Peto odds ratio', which is a particular method of calculating an odds ratio when undertaking a meta-analysis. It is an approximation of the actual odds ratio and therefore can be different from the exact odds ratio. The glossary within the database provides a useful explanation on this and many other research and statistical terms (Cochrane Collaboration 1998). You would be advised to obtain a Cochrane review and interpret the odds ratio given to confirm your understanding of this important summary statistic.

Confidence intervals are usually presented with odds ratios, so the lowest and highest OR values likely for the population are calculated from the sample data. As for all CIs the implication is that if the same study was repeated, 95% of the time the results for the repeat study would lie between the upper and lower confidence limits. If both the upper and lower CI limits are less than 1 then the treatment/care is significantly beneficial. If the CI crosses 1, then the implication is that the results are not significant, although there may be a tendency for that treatment/care to be beneficial or detrimental depending on which side of 1 the greater portion of the range between the upper and lower limits lies. The OR may be presented in graphic form, as in Figure 5.10.

The scale along the *x* axis is not necessarily linear, so the distance 0–1 is greater than the distance 1–10, and so on. The scale may be logarithmic, i.e. from 1 to 10, then 100, where the distance between 1 and 10 is the same as that between 10 and 100. This does not affect the key information being demonstrated by the graph, i.e. whether the ORs and CIs indicate beneficial or detrimental, significant or not significant outcomes. In Figure 5.10 the variables *C* and *D* are not significant but *C* has a tendency to be beneficial while *D* has a tendency to be detrimental. If both upper and lower values of the CI are greater than 1, the result is significant and detrimental, as for *B*.

The size of the range between the upper and lower confidence interval value is an indication of the amount of reliance that can be placed on the OR given. Where the range between the upper and lower confidence interval is

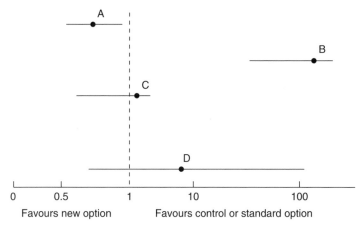

Figure 5.10 How odds ratios may be presented. The line represents the CI, the distance between the upper and lower limit, and may not be equidistant on both sides of the odds ratio point

small, for example an OR=2.0 with a CI 1.9–2.2, greater reliance can be placed on the OR than when the CI range is large, for example an OR=2.0 and a CI 0.5–5.0.

Numbers needed to treat (NNT)

The calculation of **numbers needed to treat** is a recent development, which is being encouraged by several journals, including *Evidence Based Medicine* (Evidence Based Medicine Editorial Team 1996), as it provides statistical data in a form that is readily understood by both practitioners and those they care for. It is an indication of the number of individuals who would have to be treated by the new option to prevent one adverse outcome. For example, magnesium sulphate is currently used primarily for women who have had an eclamptic fit, but there may be potential for the same drug to be used prophylactically to prevent fits in high-risk women (Eclampsia Collaborative Trial Group 1995). If this was so, an experimental study would need to evaluate the impact of prophylactic administration of magnesium sulphate on the incidence of eclamptic fits. It would then be possible to calculate the number of women who would need to be treated to prevent one fit. If 50 women need to be treated prophylactically to stop one fit, clinicians could decide whether the dangers of this drug to 49 women and the cost of administration was worth the avoidance of one fit. In addition, the 95% CI would be calculated, which would indicate the range of numbers of women that would have to be treated to prevent one fit; for this example it might be 43–57 women (these figures are for illustration only and are not based on research findings).

Absolute and relative risk reduction

The **absolute risk reduction** (ARR) is usually expressed as a percentage and indicates how many individuals less there will be with the complication or disorder if they receive the experimental treatment/management compared to if they had received the control or standard option. **Relative risk reduction** (RRR), also expressed as a percentage, is a proportion and indicates the difference between the proportion of the experimental group who had the 'condition' and the proportion in the control group who had the 'condition'. As with NNT, the aim of these statistics is to make it easier for everyone to apply and use research findings in clinical practice. As yet they are not in wide use but, as they seem to have the potential for making the interpretation of research findings from experimental studies easier, they have been included. This type of data may make informing women and their families about research findings easier and more meaningful to them.

Analysis of variance

Analysis of variance, or **ANOVA**, is a commonly used parametric test, similar to the *t* test, as it considers the significance of the difference between the means of the groups in an experimental study, using the variance as the indicator of this difference. ANOVA is used when there are three or more groups being studied. It compares the variance within groups as well as the variance between groups. If the variance between groups is significantly greater than the variance within groups, that difference is likely to be due to the different treatments of the groups. If the variance between the groups is similar to or less than the variance within groups, any differences across the groups are likely to be due to chance. There are different forms of ANOVA depending on whether the study groups are independent or matched, and a different version can be used for when there are several variables being considered across all the study groups. For information on these more complex statistical processes, please refer to one of the medical statistics texts listed.

Power calculations

A power calculation is the statistical calculation of how many participants should be included in the research study to ensure the best possibility of identifying any potential benefits or problems associated with the care or treatment under consideration. The nature and aims of the study influence sample size, and there has to be consideration of what is possible, including any clinical impact. To calculate what sample size is needed requires a knowledge of the incidence of the condition in the target population, what type of measurement level is involved, categorical or numerical, and what amount of change in that condition clinicians would consider useful or acceptable. In general, the rarer the outcome that is being measured, the larger the sample size has to be to detect a significant change. A study considering the third stage of labour would require a very large number of women if the main outcome was maternal death, a very rare event. The sample size could be fairly modest if the outcome measured was a blood loss of more than 500 ml. Power calculations are the domain of statisticians and, although computer packages are available, I would advise anyone undertaking a study to seek appropriate help. For those interested in reading further in this area, I suggest Lwanga and Lemeshow (1991).

Secondary statistical analysis

Reid (1993) suggests that secondary analysis is a nonexperimental research design and hence a valid statistical process. There is a danger of gaining misleading results from secondary analysis where the selection and allocation of the original design did not include the intention to consider the variable. This does not imply there is no value to secondary analysis: often it is the source of new insights, which can be further studied and/or generate useful debate concerning practice, but it must be made clear that this analysis is secondary and its limitations must be identified.

Systematic review and meta-analysis

A **systematic review** is the process by which all available evidence on one topic is located and evaluated to identify the best possible guide to practice. Published and unpublished sources should be included. The Centre for Reviews and Dissemination (University of York 1996) provides detailed guidance for those wishing to undertake systematic reviews and there is a comprehensive book covering the advantages, difficulties and limitations of such reviews (Chalmers and Altman 1995). This research method is the remit of skilled and experienced researchers with considerable resources at their disposal. Of these the Cochrane Collaboration is considered to provide 'the highest level of evidence ever achieved' (Sackett et al 1997, p. 15). When the systematic review includes the use of statistical methods to combine the results from several studies, it is called meta-analysis (Sackett et al 1997). This analysis takes into account the reliability and validity of the research design and sample sizes, as well as the outcomes achieved. Meta-analysis can be considered a separate research design rather than a statistical process; however I have located it here to reflect its emphasis on statistical analysis.

Further reading

There are three types of book that may be helpful for those wishing to consider statistics further. Introductory books are designed to be read through and often include examples and questions to check your understanding and to practise with. Research books include sections on statistics, in a variety of depths. These books are very useful as they provide a reference source of information that also covers explanations of other aspects of research. I would suggest that every midwife has one of these for reference. Finally, there are medical statistics books, which are of great assistance when trying to trace specific statistical tests or procedures. A list of such texts is given immediately before the references for this chapter.

CONCLUSION

This chapter has identified some of the main descriptive and inferential statistics, an understanding of which is essential in the interpretation of most quantitative research papers. While statistics can be considered a dry and difficult topic, practitioners need to recognize that they are an integral part of midwifery practice. Understanding statistical data will enable midwives to evaluate research findings and decide whether they should influence their practice. Statistics can also be used by midwives as evidence to obtain high-quality care for all women.

CHAPTER SUMMARY

This chapter has highlighted:

◆ The importance of statistics in the presentation and interpretation of research studies

◆ The main types of statistics, descriptive and inferential

◆ The most common tests, including *t* tests, chi-squared tests and tests for correlation

◆ The concept of probability and significance, along with many other statistical terms.

FURTHER READING LIST FOR STATISTICAL SUPPORT

Introductory texts
Clegg F 1982 Simple statistics. Cambridge University Press, Cambridge
Rowntree D 1981 Statistics without tears. Penguin Books, Harmondsworth

Research texts containing statistics

Hicks C M 1996 Undertaking midwifery research. A basic guide to design and analysis. Churchill Livingstone, Edinburgh

Polit D F, Hungler B P 1997 Essentials of nursing research. Methods, appraisal and utilization, 4th edn. JB Lippincott, Philadelphia, PA

Reid N 1993 Health care research by degrees. Blackwell Scientific, Oxford

Talbot L A 1995 Principles and practice of nursing research. CV Mosby, St Louis, MO

Medical statistics texts

Altman D G 1991 Practical statistics for medical research. Chapman & Hall, London

Campbell M, Machin D 1993 Medical statistics. A commonsense approach, 2nd edn. John Wiley, Chichester

Swinscow T D V 1996 Statistics at square one, 9th edn, rev Campbell M J. BMJ Publishing Group, London

REFERENCES

Altman D G 1982 Interpreting results. In: Altman D G, Gore S M Statistics in medical practice: articles published in the British Medical Journal. British Medical Association, London

Bick D E, MacArthur C 1995 Attendance, content and relevance of the six week postnatal examination. Midwifery 11(2): 69–74

Bryar R 1991 Research and individualized care in midwifery. In: Robinson S, Thomson AM (ed) Midwives, research and childbirth, vol 2. Chapman & Hall, London, ch 3, p 48–71

Campbell M J, Machin D 1993 Medical statistics. A commonsense approach, 2nd edn. John Wiley, Chichester

Chalmers I, Altman D G (ed) 1995 Systematic reviews. British Medical Journal Publishing Group, London

Clegg F 1982 Simple statistics. A course book for the social sciences. Cambridge University Press, Cambridge

Cluett E R, Alexander J, Pickering R M 1995 Is measuring the postnatal symphysis-fundal distance worthwhile? Midwifery 11(4): 174–183

Cochrane Collaboration 1998 Pregnancy and childbirth module. The Cochrane Database of Systematic Reviews. The Cochrane Collaboration: Issue 4. Update Software, Oxford

Department of Health 1993 Changing Childbirth Part 1. Report of the Expert Maternity Group. HMSO, London

Department of Health 1997 NHS maternity statistics, England: 1989–90 to 1994–95. Statistics Bulletin 28. HMSO, London

Eclampsia Collaborative Trial Group 1995 Which anticonvulsant for women with eclampsia? Evidence from the Collaborative Eclampsia Trial. Lancet 345: 1455–1463

Evidence Based Medicine Editorial Team 1996 On some clinically useful measures of the effects of treatment. Evidence Based Medicine 1(2): 37–38

Flint C, Poulengeris P, Grant A S 1989 The 'know your midwife' scheme – a randomised trial of continuity of care by a team of midwives. Midwifery 5(1): 11–16

Gore S M 1982a Assessing methods – descriptive statistics and graphs. In: Altman D G, Gore S M Statistics in medical practice: articles published in the British Medical Journal. British Medical Association, London, p 64

Gore S M 1982b Assessing methods – confidence intervals. In: Altman D G, Gore S M Statistics in medical practice: articles published in the British Medical Journal. British Medical Association, London, p 74

Hicks C M 1996 Undertaking midwifery research. A basic guide to design and analysis. Churchill Livingstone, Edinburgh

Hofmeyr G J, Nikodem V C, Wolman W-L, Chalmers B E, Kramer T 1991 Companionship to modify the clinical birth environment: effects on progress and perceptions of labour and breast feeding. British Journal of Obstetrics and Gynaecology 98(8): 756–764

Hundley V, Cruickshank F M, Lang GD et al 1994 Midwifery managed delivery unit: a randomised controlled comparison with consultant led care. British Medical Journal 309: 1400–1404

Hundley V A, Cruickshank F M, Milne J M et al 1995 Satisfaction and continuity of care: staff views of care in a midwifery managed delivery unit. Midwifery 11(4): 163–173

Johnson N, Lilford R, Guthrie K, Thornton J, Barker M, Kelly M 1997 Randomised trial comparing a policy of early with selective amniotomy in uncomplicated labour at term. British Journal of Obstetrics and Gynaecology 104(3): 340–346

Lwanga S K, Lemeshow S 1991 Sample size determination in health studies. A practice manual. World Health Organization, Geneva

Mathews F, Yudkin P, Neil A 1998 Folates in the periconceptional period: are women getting enough? British Journal of Obstetrics and Gynaecology 105(9): 954–959

Matthews J N S, Altman D G, Campbell M J, Royson P 1990 Analysis of serial measurements in medical research. British Medical Journal 300: 230–235

Polit D F, Hungler B P 1997 Essentials of nursing research. Methods, appraisal and utilization, 4th edn. JB Lippincott, Philadelphia, PA

Puri B K 1996 Statistics in practice. An illustrated guide to SPSS. Arnold Publishing. London

Reid N 1993 Health care research by degrees. Blackwell Scientific, Oxford

Roberts B L, Anthony M K, Madigan E A, Chen Y 1997 Data management: cleaning and checking. Nursing Research 46(6): 350–352

Rowntree D 1981 Statistics without tears. Penguin Books, Harmondsworth

Sackett D L, Richardson W S, Rosenberg W, Haynes R B 1997 Evidence-based medicine. How to practice and teach EBM. Churchill Livingstone, New York

Swinscow T D V 1996 Statistics at square one, 9th edn, rev Campbell, M J. British Medical Journal Publishing Group, London

University of York 1996 Undertaking systematic reviews of research on effectiveness. CRD guidelines for those carrying out or commissioning reviews. NHS Centre for Reviews and Dissemination, University of York, York

Waldenstrom U, Nilsson C-A, Winbladh B 1997 The Stockholm Birth Centre Trial: maternal and infant outcome. British Journal of Obstetrics and Gynaecology 104(4): 410–418

Wraight A, Ball J, Secombe I, Stock J 1993 Mapping team midwifery. Institute of Manpower Studies, Brighton

Wright M E 1995 A case control study of maternal nutrition and neural tube defects in Northern Ireland. Midwifery 11(3): 146–152

6

Grounded theory

Rosalind Bluff

INTRODUCTION

Grounded theory is one of the main approaches to qualitative research. This chapter will discuss the key features of grounded theory. Comparisons with quantitative research will be made to justify where the approach is placed on the quantitative/qualitative continuum. Examples of grounded theory studies relevant to midwives will be given.

Strauss (1987) suggests that grounded theory is an approach to collecting and analysing data rather than a method. Nevertheless, there is a lack of consistency in terminology. Streubert and Carpenter (1999) and Holloway and Wheeler (1996) refer to grounded theory as an approach. Strauss and Corbin (1994) use the term 'methodology' while in a subsequent text (Strauss and Corbin 1998) they emphasize grounded theory as a methodology but also refer to it as an approach and a method. No explanation is provided to account for this variation in terminology, but all agree that grounded theory enables theory to be generated from and grounded in the data through a process of data collection and analysis. Strauss and Corbin (1994, p. 275) also suggest that grounded theory is 'a way of thinking and conceptualizing the data'. For this reason it can be used by researchers in a variety of disciplines and for studies that adopt ethnographic, phenomenological and other qualitative approaches.

Holloway and Wheeler (1996) acknowledged the popularity of grounded theory among nurses, but in the last few years midwives have also begun to recognize the benefits of adopting this approach (Bluff and Holloway 1994, Walker et al 1995, Donovan 1995, Hall and Holloway 1998). Some studies such as those by Bright (1992), Beck (1993), Vasquez (1995), Barclay et al (1997) and Rogan et al (1997) explore issues related to childbirth and maternity care which are of relevance to midwives although the researchers are not themselves midwives.

ORIGINS

Glaser and Strauss (1967), both sociologists, developed the grounded theory approach in the 1960s while exploring the experiences of patients who were dying in hospital. The published results of this research (Glaser and Strauss 1965, 1968) revolutionized the way health professionals communicated with dying patients and their relatives, changing their approach from one of subterfuge to open discussion. *The Discovery of Grounded Theory* (Glaser and Strauss 1967) was published as a result of their research but it is Strauss and Corbin (1998) who provide practical guidance on how to do grounded theory.

Grounded theory is based on the beliefs of **symbolic interactionism**. Strauss was particularly influenced by interactionists such as Mead and Blumer (Strauss and Corbin 1998), who believed that the way people behaved was determined by how they interpreted their world. Within a social group, individuals have a shared understanding of what certain symbols mean to them. These are based on attitudes, values and beliefs that form part of the culture. The meaning of these symbols, which include verbal and nonverbal communications and the appearance of others, enables interpretations to be made so that people can interact with each other and their environment (Mead 1934). Individuals therefore respond to the behaviour of others and in doing so are shaped or moulded by their social environment.

This does not, however, mean that individuals passively respond to the way in which others behave. Interactionists emphasize the influence individuals have in creating their own social environment through actively participating in their surroundings. For example, women who are in labour have a need for information. When questions go unanswered they develop specific strategies to enable them to obtain the information they want. These include 'eavesdropping' on conversations when midwives are teaching students and the use of 'self-denigration', which midwives always respond to (Kirkham 1987). Grounded theory therefore seeks to identify the processes that explain what is happening in a social setting. This is achieved by exploring how people behave from a symbolic and interactional perspective. By uncovering the symbols or shared understandings that enable individuals to interpret their world, grounded theory makes explicit the social processes of interaction that individuals within a culture implicitly know but those outside the culture do not. Because the way individuals behave is influenced by their environment, it is important that the context in which a grounded theory study takes place should be described and taken into account when analysing the data (Morse and Field 1996).

For the purposes of this book, grounded theory has been placed in the middle of the quantitative/qualitative continuum illustrated in Chapter 2. According to Strauss and Corbin (1998) Glaser was influenced by Paul Lazarsfield, who specialized in quantitative research methods. It may be because of this that grounded theory has a number of features associated with quantitative research. The terms used in their original text (Glaser and Strauss 1967) to express their ideas, such as 'precision', 'hypotheses' and 'variables' appear to have originated from the quantitative paradigm. This may be related to its origins or alternatively may have been because the book was written when qualitative research was not considered trustworthy and the language of quantitative research made it more acceptable.

Qualitative research is a dynamic process. An approach to research developed using sociological data is unlikely to meet all the needs of practitioners working in the health-care setting. Most researchers therefore have a need to adapt the approach to meet the needs of a study undertaken in the context of their own discipline. In this way, an approach evolves over a period of time. Indeed, Strauss and Corbin (1994) believe that grounded theory will evolve as more researchers use the approach to study an increasing variety of phenomena. Glaser (1992), however, is adamant that since its inception grounded theory has been eroded by Strauss. Stern (1994) points out that the approaches they adopted always were different. This was recognized by their students but not by Glaser until the publication of Strauss and Corbin 1990.

PURPOSES

Grounded theory is a creative process that facilitates the development of new theory (Strauss and Corbin 1998). For this reason it is an appropriate approach to use when there is a lack of knowledge about a topic (Glaser and Strauss 1967, Stern 1980). A grounded theory study is valuable in its own right but in these circumstances, if considered appropriate, the results can also be used to inform a large quantitative study, the findings of which can then be generalized to a population. Bluff (ongoing study) adopted a grounded theory approach to explore the midwife as a role model because, as Stern (1980) suggests, it is appropriate when the topic has been investigated by others but not by one's own discipline. Beck's (1993) justification for the use of grounded theory when developing her theory of postpartum depression was to adopt a new perspective on a topic that had mainly been investigated using quantitative research approaches. On completion of this study the findings were compared with those of a phenomenological study on the same topic. In doing so, existing theory was modified and extended. This supports the views of Strauss and Corbin (1998) that grounded theories should not be viewed in isolation but compared with others in the same field of study. Hutchinson (1986) also believes that grounded theory is useful for clarifying existing theory.

As midwives seek to fulfil the requirements of the Department of Health's report (Department of Health 1993) and provide care that meets women's needs, grounded theory provides one valuable means of ascertaining women's perspective on midwifery and maternity care. The perspective of midwives, students and others who provide that care can also be obtained. How women interact with their carers and indeed how their carers interact with them and other members of the health-care team can influence the quality of care that is received (Kirkham 1987). What influences these interactions is therefore important. Grounded theory studies may be helpful in ascertaining the effects of the introduction of primary care groups (Department of Health 1997) on midwives, consumers and the way in which maternity care is organized. Streubert and Carpenter (1999) also consider grounded theory to be an appropriate approach for researching issues related to education and management.

FEATURES OF GROUNDED THEORY

A number of features are associated specifically with grounded theory. We noted in Chapter 2 that qualitative research is generally regarded as being **inductive** (Leininger 1985), meaning that theory is generated from the data. This differs from quantitative research, where one begins with a theory or hypothesis, which is tested and subsequently accepted or rejected. Grounded theory is, however, both inductive and **deductive** (Glaser and Strauss 1967, Stern 1980, Strauss and Corbin 1998). As the theory emerges from the data, working hypotheses are formulated. These are tested as further data are collected. For example, it became evident when exploring women's experiences of labour and birth (Bluff and Holloway 1994) that women in the lower socioeconomic groups perceived that health professionals knew what care was best for them. The working hypothesis or proposition that middle class women would be less likely to accept that professionals knew what care was best for them was tested and rejected.

Sample

The sample size in a grounded theory study tends to be small, as it does in most qualitative research studies. Hall and Holloway (1998) included nine women in their study of women's experiences of labouring in water. Morse and Johnson (1991) identify four qualities that participants need to have for inclusion in a grounded theory study, although it could be argued that these qualities equally apply to participants in any type of qualitative research study (Box 6.1).

Box 6.1 Qualities necessary for participation in a grounded theory study (Morse and Johnson 1991)

◆ Participants must have knowledge of the phenomenon that is being studied. For this reason, the sample is called a **purposive** or purposeful one
◆ Participants must be willing to participate
◆ Participants must have the time to participate
◆ Individuals need to be articulate in expressing their views

---

For theory to be developed, the quality of data collected is important. There is, however, the danger of biasing the sample, for example, in favour of those in the upper socioeconomic groups. Everyone has their story to tell and, although the quality of data obtained from those who are less articulate may be poor, data from these participants may be sufficient to confirm or refute the findings of others. If the data is not sufficient to achieve this, it cannot contribute to the development of a theory and therefore cannot be used.

The sample that is selected will have a major influence on the theory that is developed. Sampling is therefore an important issue and needs to be considered prior to commencement of the study. Sample size is, however, determined by theoretical **saturation** of categories, and which individuals are sampled is influenced by analysis of the data. For this reason, sampling will be returned to when these issues are addressed.

Data collection

Data may be collected in a number of ways. In order to learn about women's experiences of birth, Bluff and Holloway (1994) collected data by means of interviews, which were tape-recorded. If you are going to use a tape recorder, do remember to check that your equipment works prior to the event. It is also helpful to have with you both batteries and a transformer. Should the batteries fail, you will then have an alternative energy supply.

Interviews enable the researcher to obtain information in the participant's own words. Open-ended questions provide participants with the opportunity to talk freely about the issues that are important to them. This helps researchers to avoid imposing their own ideas on the study. **Unstructured interviews** are usually associated with one or two open-ended questions. However, as the theory emerges from the data, data collection becomes more focused and is modified to enable the researcher to concentrate on those issues that will facilitate the development of a theory that is **conceptually dense** (May 1991). By this, Strauss and Corbin (1994) mean the development of a theory in which concepts are clearly related to each other and numerous variations in the phenomenon are identified. For this reason, interviews are usually **semistructured** or become so as the study progresses. Researchers often find an interview guide listing key concepts helpful in reminding them of issues that need to be addressed (Hutchinson 1986). A wide range of data that has depth and detail can be collected when the interview is allowed to proceed like a conversation, with issues being discussed as they arise (Couchman and Dawson 1995).

If concepts of importance to the developing theory are not mentioned by participants the researcher can ask questions to obtain their views. Do be careful to avoid asking leading questions, as participants' answers will be a response to your own preconceived ideas and not necessarily an indication of their views or opinions. This approach to interviewing does sometimes result in issues emerging that the researcher might not otherwise have thought of.

Data can also be collected by observing situations and events. In grounded theory studies this is often the favoured strategy for collecting data because it enables interactions of individuals with others and their environment to be witnessed and interpreted. Participant observation requires the researcher to fulfil a role within the environment in which the study takes place while observing participants. Nonparticipant observation corresponds to the 'fly on the wall' and the dilemmas associated with this approach have been addressed by Kirkham (1987). Methods of data collection are frequently combined. Bowler (1993) chose nonparticipant observation and interviewing as the preferred methods of data collection, while Bright (1992) and Beck (1993) opted for participant observation in combination with interviews. This combination of data collection methods can help to verify the truth of the data. What is said to the researcher is not necessarily what is done in practice.

A variety of sources can be used for data collection (Strauss and Corbin 1994; Box 6.2). Videotapes can also be used to record observations and interactions of people but care must be taken to address the ethical issues.

Box 6.2 Sources of data for use in a grounded theory study

◆ Women's maternity care notes
◆ Letters
◆ Off-duty rotas
◆ Hospital and community trust policies
◆ Protocols
◆ Guidelines
◆ Diaries completed by participants
◆ Other relevant documents

To enhance all methods of data collection, **field notes** can be kept. In this way the context in which the research took place and aspects of nonverbal communication are recorded. Field notes are particularly important when gathering data by observation, as this may be the only means of recording data (Morse and Field 1996).

It is important to be aware that in any qualitative study the researcher is the research tool and therefore becomes a part of the research study. Because of this the researcher may unknowingly influence participants and the data collected. Hutchinson (1986) recommends that researchers keep a reflective diary so they are aware of the effect they may have on participants and the data that are collected. In this way, researchers can reflect on how they may have influenced participants, or indeed how participants may have influenced them, and the effect that this has had on their study. Researchers can reflect on their experience of the research process or their experiences in relation to the topic under investigation. They may also identify pre-existing ideas, values and beliefs (Hutchinson 1986). The issue of a reflective diary is addressed in greater detail in Chapter 7.

Data analysis

Before data can be analysed it must first be transcribed. This means that observations and data obtained during interviews are recorded in writing, word for word. Remember that your transcript will also need to record coughs, laughs, pauses and gestures, as these can all influence your interpretation of the data. Holloway (1997) and Morse and Field (1996) provide practical detail of what transcribing entails.

Data are analysed by means of the **constant comparative method**, in which the collection and analysis of data is a parallel process (Glaser and Strauss 1967). Data are therefore collected and analysed and the process is repeated as often as necessary. From a very early stage in the research process, concepts within the data are identified. Open coding involves naming incidents, ideas and events to give meaning to the data (Strauss and Corbin 1998). These substantive codes, so called because they come from the substance of the data, may be 'in vivo', i.e. words that the participants themselves have used, or may be words identified by the researcher that give meaning to the data. Hutchinson (1986) calls these level 1 codes. In this way, questions are generated from the data and one incident is compared with another. Each interview or set of data is compared and as new ideas emerge further comparisons are made. You may find it helpful to record the data on one half of the paper so that codes appear next to the data to which they are related, as illustrated in Table 6.1.

Table 6.1 Conceptualizing the data

Interview data	Open Coding
Um, people would ask me to get things and I wouldn't know where they were. I would try and find where things were but things would happen so quickly and you're expected to run around and get things. I just felt like an outsider. I went into the office on the very first day. I'd got my uniform on and nobody really said oh welcome and I just sat there thinking what am I doing here. So I was at that stage on that ward that I didn't know whether I wanted to carry on. It was that bad, the stress.	lack of knowledge trying to help skivvy outsider (in vivo code) beginner ignored, lack of professional identity experiencing doubt experiencing doubt stressed

The use of this method of analysis enables a considerable number of concepts to emerge from the data. Similar concepts are linked together to form categories or level 2 codes (Hutchinson 1986), thus providing order for the data. These categories are renamed to achieve a higher level of abstraction. For example concepts entitled 'trust', 'acceptance', 'blind faith' emerging from interviews formed a category which was named 'they know best' (Bluff and Holloway 1994). Further linking and reduction of the number of these categories to form major categories produces what Hutchinson (1986) calls level 3 codes. **Axial coding** (Strauss and Corbin 1998) enables categories to be connected to each other by identifying such issues as the context and conditions under which a phenomenon occurs and the consequences associated with its occurrence. A process of **selective coding** (Strauss and Corbin 1998) facilitates the emergence of a **core category** or story line. The core category is related to all other categories and provides an explanation of how people behave in a particular social environment. Just as concepts emerge from the data, so too should the theory. Beck (1993) provides an excellent illustration of the different levels of code.

The core category

The core category or story line is the central or main theme that emerges from the data. It explains what is happening in the social setting but may only become apparent as the study draws to an end (Strauss 1987). Other features are also associated with this core category (Strauss 1987). It occurs frequently in the data and links all other data together. Variation in the data is also explained by the core category. This variation contributes to the conceptual density of the theory, which is developed and occurs because few individuals or cases exactly match the central theme (Strauss and Corbin 1998).

The core category or social process that emerged from Beck's (1993) study was that women who suffered from postnatal depression experienced a loss of control so strong that they hovered between sanity and insanity. Further understanding of this process was achieved by the development of subcategories that identified the strategies women adopted to cope with their perceived loss of control. The process of linking and reducing categories can result in what Lofland and Lofland (1984, p. 138) call the 'agony of omission'. This means that information or concepts that the researcher wishes to convey to others has to be omitted from the final write up of the report because it does not fit in with the story line (Glaser 1978). Such information should not, however, be disregarded, because it is important to the participants who wanted to tell their story. Time permitting, it provides the researcher with ample opportunity to write further articles for publication.

According to Strauss and Corbin (1998), there are clear ways of going about grounded theory and the detailed and systematic way of doing this might be perceived to be prescriptive. Strauss (1987) does, however, argue that while specific procedures should be followed there must also be some flexibility. The ability to cope with ambiguity is an advantage (Glesne and Peshkin 1992). It is only when the relationship between codes and categories becomes clear that the story line emerges. Until then the researcher is faced with numerous codes, which appear to bear no relationship to each other. Unaware of the final outcome of the study the researcher is constantly 'leaping in the dark'. This can be frustrating and at times disheartening. However, it is important to relax and believe in the process, because ultimately relationships do become apparent. It can be particularly helpful at this stage to discuss your research with colleagues. The verbal expression of your findings can stimulate questions and ideas which, when shared with the thoughts of your colleagues, may enhance your understanding.

Theoretical saturation

Theoretical saturation of categories is said to have been achieved when no new data about those categories emerges during further data collection and analysis (Strauss and Corbin 1998). Modification of the interview content continues until all theoretical categories have been saturated (Glaser and Strauss 1967). Dreher (1994) argues that, in achieving saturation of categories, qualitative researchers focus on the amount or quantity of data related to each aspect of the phenomenon under study. This corresponds to the quantitative researcher's concern for amount and measurement of data. Dreher (1994) does, however, warn of the danger of focusing on collecting data until saturation is achieved. Through doing so, she believes, other concepts or categories of importance may not emerge and be discussed. No explanation is offered for this belief but it is possible that the preoccupation with achieving saturation of specific categories may preclude the researcher from asking questions that would facilitate the emergence of other issues.

The number of participants in a grounded theory study is determined by the theoretical saturation of each category (Glaser and Strauss 1967) and is not known in advance. Morse and Johnson (1991) acknowledge that, when some participants are less articulate, the sample size may need to be larger to achieve saturation and this has implications for researchers who have a limited time in which to complete their study.

Memos and diagrams

Abstract thinking about the data is recorded in the form of **memos** (Strauss and Corbin 1998). This provides a means of organizing and controlling the data. As the theory develops, these memos become more detailed and form the basis from which the final report is written. Each memo may record areas of thinking or conceptualization of the data, questions that are raised as a result of this process, the formulation of hypotheses and ideas on how concepts are related to each other (Strauss and Corbin 1998). Writing memos is a continual process throughout the study and what is written in them forms a major contribution to the development of theory. The memo illustrated in Box 6.3 provides a record of thoughts and questions raised by the data presented in Table 6.1.

> **Box 6.3** Memo extrapolating from interview data
>
> Sandy is a junior student on her first clinical placement in the maternity unit. She lacks knowledge of the clinical environment but tries to help the midwives she works with when they ask her to get things for them. It appears that circumstances change quickly and the midwives need a 'skivvy'. This raises a number of questions. Is it appropriate for the student to fulfil this role? If it is simply a case of getting essential items for the midwife could this role be fulfilled by a health-care assistant? What learning opportunities does the student miss while she fulfils the role of a handmaiden?
>
> On the first day of this placement the student appears to feel excluded. Although she is wearing the uniform of a student, the midwives do not know her and she lacks a professional identity. This may explain why Sandy's presence is not acknowledged. Such behaviour, however, might be described as rude and discourteous. Little wonder that Sandy feels stressed and begins to doubt her decision to be a midwife.

Memos can be written about each concept. As more data is collected and analysed these can be revised. When relationships between codes and concepts have been identified and the number reduced to form categories, the contents of a number of memos can be amalgamated, revised and recorded under the title of the category. This approach to collecting, analysing and recording data can result in the production of an enormous number of words. Morse (1993) warns that the researcher should not drown in the data. Nevertheless, a feeling of drowning may be encountered by the inexperienced grounded theorist.

The relationship between codes and categories can also be visually represented in the form of diagrams. Beck (1993) provides a good example of this. These have the advantage of graphically displaying the content of memos in a clear and concise manner and may identify where gaps in knowledge still exist and further data needs to be collected (Strauss and Corbin 1998).

Theoretical sampling

In the initial stages of the study, when the relevance of data is not known, Strauss and Corbin (1998) recommend **open sampling**. This means that the researcher is open to interviewing any participant, observing any events or examining any documents that might provide data of interest to the study. As important issues emerge, **theoretical sampling** takes priority. This type of sampling facilitates the development of theory by enabling new participants to be sought in response to analysis of the data. On occasions it may not be possible to theoretically sample individuals. Concepts can, however, be sampled in this way by questioning individuals about an issue if they do not spontaneously talk about the topic themselves. The emerging theory therefore controls the collection of data (Glaser and Strauss 1967). Bluff and Holloway (1994), for example, identified that primigravid women believed that health professionals knew what care was best for them. This finding led the researchers to sample multigravid women to identify whether they too held the same belief. In this way concepts and categories can be confirmed, rejected or extended (Strauss and Corbin 1998). Participants who will support and refute the concepts and categories or are likely to have a different perspective on events are deliberately sought (Strauss and Corbin 1998). In this way, a theory that is conceptually dense and well integrated is developed. It is important to remember that the relationship between data collection and analysis is crucial. If all data are collected first, answers to questions generated from the data may not be answered and theoretical sampling will not occur unless the analyst is doing some analysis in her/his head.

Theoretical sensitivity

Theoretical sensitivity is an essential requirement for the development of a theory that is grounded in the data. By this Glaser and Strauss (1967) mean that researchers must have the ability to immerse themselves in the data and give meaning to it. The ability to recognize what data are relevant to the emerging theory is therefore an essential requirement. One could argue that sensitivity is a necessary requisite for the analysis of all qualitative data. While this is true, sensitivity for ethnographers and phenomenologists is to the meaning and interpretation of data rather than the development of a theory, which is sought by grounded theorists.

Personal and professional knowledge and experience can enhance the researcher's sensitivity to the data (Strauss and Corbin 1998). Alternatively, it may prove to be a disadvantage. The existence of preconceived ideas associated with familiarity with the data, unless acknowledged, may reduce the researcher's sensitivity. Whatever the effects researchers may have, these should be made explicit in the study. A good command of the English language facilitates the naming of codes and categories and thus enhances theoretical sensitivity. For this reason, a thesaurus may be an essential item for some grounded theorists.

Theoretical sensitivity may also be enhanced by appropriate use of available literature (Glaser 1978). The consistent presence of concepts in published literature may increase the researcher's ability to recognize these concepts in their own data or in their absence to ask questions of future participants to ascertain why they are absent (Strauss and Corbin 1998).

Using the literature

A detailed initial literature review is considered inappropriate (Glaser and Strauss 1967, Strauss and Corbin 1998) because of the risk of developing preconceived ideas that may inhibit the development of a theory. Completion of a research proposal does, however, warrant some form of literature review (Chenitz and Swanson 1986) and advantages can be gained from this undertaking. A general overview of the available literature enables any qualitative researcher to justify her/his chosen approach (De Poy and Gitlin 1993) and avoids the possibility of replicating studies. Morse and Johnson (1991), however, specify the need to put to one side the knowledge gained from this procedure in order to avoid influencing data collection. You may question whether this can realistically be achieved. Identifying what is or is not known about a topic also enables researchers to refine the area of their study (Glesne and Peshkin 1992). The importance of the topic area and how the findings of their study will add to the body of knowledge can also be identified (Chenitz and Swanson 1986).

Although the initial literature review is limited, reference to the literature continues throughout the research study. This means that ultimately the literature is extensively reviewed. As findings emerge, these are compared with what is already known on the subject (Strauss and Corbin 1998, Morse and Johnson 1991). Available evidence may support the researcher's findings. Where disagreement exists, the reasons for this are explored. The literature therefore generates questions that influence subsequent data collection. In this way, the literature becomes incorporated into the data. Reference to the literature also enables the researcher to view the phenomenon from the perspective of other disciplines or social contexts and in this way extend her/his theory.

The theory

According to Strauss and Corbin (1994) the main difference between grounded theory and other qualitative approaches is the importance that is placed on the development of theory. It is the process of data collection and analysis that enables the theory to emerge from the data. This is developed, refined and verified (Strauss and Corbin 1998). This verification can only be provisional. The social environment is dynamic and theories are likely to be refined or modified in response to contextual changes (Strauss and Corbin 1994). Despite this, theory that is grounded in the data will, according to Glaser and Strauss (1967), continue to be relevant. Their theory of patients dying in hospital continues to influence the practice of health carers in the late 1990s.

A grounded theory can be recognized as good when it meets the criteria of fit, understanding, generality, and control (Glaser and Strauss 1967). A theory is said to *fit* when it is recognized as representing the reality of all those who are involved in the area of study. This might include pregnant women and the midwives and students who care for them. For this reason, the theory is *understood* by those individuals and because of its relevance to them it has credibility. It is important to remember that individuals' view of reality will vary and will in part be dependent upon past experiences and the setting in which the phenomenon is explored. If, however, the theory is conceptually dense, Glaser and Strauss (1967) believe that the theory will achieve a level of abstraction that enables it to be applied in other contexts where the phenomenon that was studied can be found. Hence its **generality**, although Lincoln and Guba (1985) prefer to use the term 'transferability'. The theory should also offer *control*. In other words, as midwifery practitioners we should have the autonomy to use the theory and adjust it to the prevailing circumstances or in response to the effects or consequences it has on the mothers and babies we care for.

Hutchinson (1986) acknowledges that on occasions a theory may lack completeness. This often occurs because saturation of codes and theoretical categories has not been achieved. Time constraints associated with undertaking a grounded theory study for a first- or second-level degree may sometimes account for this. Therefore it may be appropriate to consider an alternative approach if your time is limited. A lack of understanding of the approach can result in conceptualizing or coding the data, but without theoretical sampling the theory lacks density (Glaser and Strauss 1967). Glaser and Strauss (1967) also suggest that some researchers use procedures associated with grounded theory when they have no intention of developing theory. Kirkham (1987), in an ethnographic study, chose to make comparisons of interactions between midwives, pregnant women and doctors in different settings where women gave birth. Such comparisons as we have seen are a feature of grounded theory. Ethnography is not commonly associated with these comparisons, nor is there an intention to develop theory. What Kirkham (1987) provides is a descriptive study. Researchers may be faced with a dilemma if a core category does not emerge from the data, because without it they lack a theory (Hutchinson

1986). Faced with this situation Hutchinson (1986) suggests that the study may be presented as a descriptive one.

ETHICAL ISSUES

Glaser and Strauss (1967) and Strauss and Corbin (1998) make no reference to ethical issues associated with grounded theory. Nevertheless they cannot be ignored. The ethical issues that need to be considered apply to all qualitative approaches and are not unique to grounded theory. Approval from the appropriate Ethics Committee must be sought to undertake any research that involves the participation of clients. Access to the setting has to be gained via **gate-keepers** (Morse and Field 1996). Confidentiality and anonymity must be maintained. This can create dilemmas, particularly when the sample size is small. Documentation in the form of text, tapes and video recordings must be carefully stored with no identifying features. The need for informed consent raises particular issues, as does the issue of the researcher's influence on the participants and the data. Readers need to refer to other texts, such as Holloway and Wheeler 1996 and Ramos 1989 for more detailed information on these and other issues. You will find that some texts encompass ethics in relation to quantitative as well as qualitative research. Ramos (1989) notes that ethical standards related to quantitative research are usually generalized to the qualitative paradigm. You will therefore need to have a clear understanding of the approach and the method involved when interpreting and applying ethical issues to grounded theory and other qualitative approaches.

CONCLUSION

Grounded theory is a qualitative approach to collecting and analysing the data, the purpose of which is to develop a conceptually dense theory that explains what is happening in the social setting. Although a qualitative approach, many of its features can be compared to the quantitative research process. I know from my own experience that grounded theory can be a very laborious and time-consuming process. According to Strauss (1987) it can be both 'boring' and 'exciting'. Like all qualitative research, grounded theory is a process of discovery. The emergence of a theory and the serendipity associated with this type of research provides ample reward for the committed researcher.

CHAPTER SUMMARY

This chapter has highlighted that:

Grounded theory is an approach to collecting and analysing data.

The process involves:

◆ a small literature review to justify the study

◆ an ongoing purposive sample

◆ data collection using unstructured and semistructured interviews

◆ observation of events

◆ written documents

◆ the constant comparative method of analysis

◆ theoretical sampling and sensitivity

◆ saturation of theoretical categories

◆ incorporating literature into the data

It is a detailed and systematic approach that enables theory to be developed.

Grounded theory can enable midwives to interpret how people behave and how that behaviour is influenced by interaction with others and their environment.

REFERENCES

Barclay L, Everitt L, Rogan F, Schmied V, Wyllie A 1997 Becoming a mother – an analysis of women's experience of early motherhood. Journal of Advanced Nursing 25(4): 719–728

Beck C T 1993 Teetering on the edge: a substantive theory of postnatal depression. Nursing Research 42(1): 42–48

Bluff R Ongoing study. Fitting in and staying out of trouble: the influence of midwives on student learning

Bluff R, Holloway I 1994 'They know best': women's perceptions of midwifery care during labour and childbirth. Midwifery 10(3): 157–164

Bowler I 1993 'They're not the same as us': midwives' stereotypes of South Asian descent maternity patients. Sociology of Health and Illness 15(2): 157–177

Bright A O 1992 Making place: the first birth in an intergenerational family context. Qualitative Health Research 2(1): 75–98

Chenitz W C, Swanson J M 1986 From practice to grounded theory: qualitative research in nursing. Addison Wesley, Menlo Park, CA

Couchman W, Dawson J 1995 Nursing and health-care research: a practical guide. Scutari Press, London

De Poy E, Gitlin L N 1993 Introduction to research: multiple strategies for health and human sciences. Mosby, St Louis, MO

Department of Health 1993 Changing childbirth. Report of the Expert Maternity Group. HMSO, London

Department of Health 1997 The new NHS: modern, dependable. London, HMSO

Donovan J 1995 The process of analysis during a grounded theory study of men during their partners' pregnancies. Journal of Advanced Nursing 21(4): 708–715

Dreher M 1994 Qualitative research methods from the reviewer's perspective. In: Morse J M (ed) Critical issues in qualitative research methods. Sage Publications, Thousand Oaks, CA, ch 15, p 281–297

Glaser B G 1978 Theoretical sensitivity. Sociology Press, Mill Valley, CA

Glaser B G 1992 Basics of grounded theory analysis. Sociology Press, Mill Valley, CA

Glaser B, Strauss A 1965 Awareness of dying. Aldine Press, Chicago, IL

Glaser B G, Strauss A L 1967 The discovery of grounded theory: strategies for qualitative research. Aldine De Gruyter, New York

Glaser B, Strauss A 1968 Time for dying. Aldine Press, Chicago, IL

Glesne C, Peshkin A 1992 Becoming qualitative researchers: an introduction. Longman, New York

Hall S M, Holloway I M 1998 Staying in control: women's experiences of labour in water. Midwifery 14(1): 30–36

Holloway I 1997 Basic concepts for qualitative research. Blackwell Science, Oxford

Holloway I, Wheeler S 1996 Qualitative research for nurses. Blackwell Science, Oxford

Hutchinson S 1986 Grounded theory: the method. In: Munhall P L, Oiler C J (ed) Nursing research: a qualitative perspective. Appleton-Century-Crofts, Norwalk, CT, ch 6, p 111–130

Kirkham M 1987 Basic supportive care in labour: interaction with and around women in labour. PhD thesis, University of Manchester

Leininger M M 1985 Qualitative research methods in nursing. Grune & Stratton, Orlando, FL

Lincoln Y S, Guba E G 1985 Naturalistic inquiry. Sage Publications, Newbury Park, CA

Lofland J, Lofland L H 1984 Analyzing social settings: a guide to qualitative observation and analysis. Wadsworth, Belmont, CA

May K A 1991 Interview techniques in qualitative research: concerns and challenges. In: Morse J (ed) Qualitative nursing research – a contemporary dialogue. Sage Publications, London, ch 11, p 188–201

Mead G H 1934 Mind, self and society. University of Chicago Press, Chicago, IL

Morse J M 1993 Drowning in data. Qualitative Health Research 3(3): 267–269

Morse J M, Field P A 1996 Nursing research: the application of qualitative approaches. Chapman & Hall, London

Morse J M, Johnson J L 1991 Understanding the illness experience. In: Morse J M, Johnson J L The illness experience: dimensions of suffering. Sage Publications, Newbury Park, CA, ch 1, p 1–12

Ramos M C 1989 Some ethical implications of qualitative research. Research in Nursing and Health 12: 57–63

Rogan F, Shmied V, Barclay L, Everitt L, Wyllie A 1997 'Becoming a mother' – developing a new theory of early motherhood. Journal of Advanced Nursing 25(5): 877–885

Stern P N 1980 Grounded theory methodology. Its uses and processes. Image 12: 20–23

Stern P N 1994 Eroding grounded theory. In: Morse J M (ed) Critical issues on qualitative research methods. Sage Publications, Thousand Oaks, CA, ch 11, p 212–223

Strauss A L 1987 Qualitative analysis for social scientists. Cambridge University Press, Cambridge

Strauss A, Corbin J 1990 Basics of qualitative research grounded theory procedures and techniques. Sage Publications, Newbury Park

Strauss A, Corbin J 1994 Grounded theory methodology: an overview. In: Denzin N K, Lincoln Y S (ed) Handbook of qualitative research. Sage Publications, London, ch 17, p 273–285

Strauss A, Corbin J 1998 Basics of qualitative research techniques and procedures for developing grounded theory, 2nd edn. Sage Publications, Thousand Oaks, CA

Streubert H J, Carpenter D R 1999 Qualitative research in nursing: advancing the humanistic imperative, 2nd edn. JB Lippincott, Philadelphia, PA

Vasquez E 1995 Creating paths: living with a very-low-birth-weight infant. Journal of Obstetric, Gynecologic and Neonatal Nursing 24(8): 619–624

Walker J M, Hall S, Thomas M 1995 The experience of labour: a perspective from those receiving care in a midwife-led unit. Midwifery 11(3): 120–129

7

Ethnography

Patricia Donovan

INTRODUCTION

'Pregnancy and childbirth are social events in that they take place within a surrounding economic and social system and are understood within a cultural value system' (Symonds and Hunt 1996, p. 83).

Ethnography and ethnographic data can expose the hidden cultural contexts of childbirth, motherhood and the life of women to the world at large. This may be helpful to midwives, who may have only seen them from their own perspective. Through ethnography, midwives can understand pregnancy, childbirth and motherhood from a cultural perspective as well as demonstrate knowledge of the physiological processes that take place. This understanding can lead to quality care for women and influence policy (Silverman 1993). Feminist ethnographers would suggest that ethnography and the whole area of qualitative research gives voice to the hitherto hidden and silent voice of women in society.

Ethnography is a means of obtaining a holistic view of people in their physical and sociocultural environment and making some sense of their behaviour and interactions within that setting. Werner and Schoepfle (1987) explain that ethnography is any full or partial description of a group, *ethno-* meaning 'folk' and *graphy* meaning 'description'; therefore 'a description of folk'. There is disagreement in sociological literature about a precise definition of ethnography and the differences between ethnography and other qualitative research methods. Differences may be due to the perspective of the researcher. Ethnography can be seen as an approach that may include other methods of data analysis, such as those adopted by phenomenologists and grounded theorists. Hunt and Symonds (1995), in their discussion of the culture of the labour ward, discuss the confusion regarding grounded theory and ethnography but do not offer any further clarification. This chapter will explore ethnography as a separate entity while acknowledging that there are areas of overlap and disagreement with other research approaches (Morse and Field 1996).

ORIGINS

Historically, ethnography has evolved from within cultural anthropology. It has been used as a research approach since the early 20th century, with the works of Frank Boas (1924) and Margaret Mead (1929), and is the principal method by which anthropologists have studied previously unknown and normally primitive tribes and societies. It is based on the premise that all humans share sufficient characteristics in common to begin to develop social relationships. This is also a premise on which midwifery is based, as it assumes that women have common attributes and characteristics that enable relationships to be established.

As the number of unknown societies has diminished, anthropologists have sought other societies to study and they have been joined by educationalists, sociologists and health professionals as they endeavour to make sense of subcultures and groups within society.

PURPOSE

The ethnographer attempts to discover what is happening and how it is happening, and to offer meaning or some form of interpretation (Leininger 1985). Ethnography endeavours to act as an intelligent camera, not only allowing the reader of ethnographic studies to see the interactions and behaviour of a culture but also to instil some sense of meaning into an otherwise strange or even familiar behaviour. It endeavours to get 'inside the skin' of those being studied. For this reason, ethnography can be seen as subjective, but it makes no excuses for this. Ethnography is naturalistic, as it examines interactions within their natural settings and environment. Like all research, it is concerned with discovery and ethnographers find it 'an exciting enterprise on which to embark' (Davies 1985, p. 224).

Box 7.1 Types of ethnography

◆ **Classical ethnography** is a product of prolonged contact with a group. The researcher studies, documents and participates in specific activity.

◆ **Systematic ethnography** attempts to define and delineate a specific cultural structure. It seeks to provide meaning for the behaviour observed, allowing understanding of motivational factors. This may also be called cognitive ethnography. It focuses on methods related to data collection and analysis.

◆ **Interpretive ethnography** attempts to discover the meanings of social interaction and behaviour and focuses on the analytical and interpretive processes. This is accomplished by depicting behaviour in terms of the culture in which it occurs (Jacobson 1991).

◆ **Critical ethnography** emphasizes the subjectivity of the researcher and how the researcher is instrumental in data collection. It explores the values of the researcher and takes them into account during the analysis of the data.

It is only recently that midwives have seen ethnography as a valid research approach to explore the culture of childbirth within the UK, whereas it has been used by sociologists and anthropologists to study the role of childbirth and women within societies (Jordan 1980). In the MIRIAD database there are only a small percentage of studies that have used an ethnographic approach. This may be because the majority of midwives are women and they may already have ascribed meaning to childbirth and not seen the culture as strange. Whatever the reason, ethnography can bring a new understanding to midwives' work, such as that of Kirkham (1987) and Hunt and Symonds (1995). Kirkham (1994) sees midwifery skills, such as listening and observing, as essential skills for ethnographers. Midwives whose philosophy is to observe the natural course of pregnancy and labour and take a supportive or non-participative role may have skills that can be utilized during the course of an ethnographic study. Lipson (1991), however, suggests that a good clinician does not necessarily make a good ethnographer. Midwives who prefer an active role during the process of birth and find the intensive nature of high-risk labour satisfying may find the observational skills required and the lack of participation within the field too frustrating. They therefore may choose a more quantitative approach.

Ethnography is a blanket term that includes several variations, which are described by Muecke (1994) and are identified in Box 7.1.

CHARACTERISTICS OF THE APPROACH

Boyle (1994) states that some ethnographers may emphasize specific characteristics over others but generally there is agreement that the following characteristics are displayed:

◆ the holistic and contextual nature
◆ reflexivity
◆ use of emic and etic data
◆ the end product is ethnography.

The holistic and contextual nature

Ethnographers believe that the behaviour of people can only be understood within the context in which it takes place. This includes the physical and social environment, for example Ball's study of a school (1993) and Silverman's study of a paediatric clinic (1993). The researcher acts as an observer to understand behaviour within a specific social setting.

Reflexivity

The ethnographer is part of the research process and plays a dominant role in data collection. The research process demands a certain degree of introspection, self-awareness and self-analysis by the researcher, as data is interpreted through the mind of the researcher as well as the informant. Davies (1985) puts forward the interesting analogy of the ethnographer as a form of tea strainer, decisive about the interpretation of the tea leaves but with little effect on the brew poured in. Ethnographers need to cultivate self-awareness, being aware of how they behave, both verbally and nonverbally, and how their own emotions and reactions impact on the data gathering and analysis process (Lipson 1991).

Prior to entering the field the researcher's role must be constructed carefully and is called the persona. In midwifery research it is less likely that a persona is needed, because of the overt nature of the study, unlike some sociological studies, where the researcher adopts a role within the society. An example of this can be seen in Davies's study (1996), which explored the experiences of student midwives in the initial weeks of their course. She adopted the role of a mature student and dressed accordingly to 'fit in' (Davies 1996). This could be described as a studied presentation of 'self' and has been likened to going on a 'blind date' (Ball 1993) – a personal confrontation with the unknown.

The researcher has to function effectively within the research setting. To achieve this, a rapport needs to be established with the actors, participants or informants within the field. Decisions will have to be made about whom to talk to, where to be and what relationships to establish. As data gatherer, the researcher needs to decide what should be said and done next in order to elicit more data. This balancing of the need to be part of the group and yet obtain the required data is called the integration of the subject with the object. It can be considered on a continuum of participation, from no participation to full participation.

Researchers should attempt to analyse what they hear and what they say and weigh the impact of their presence on the data gathered. They should also be aware of informants' perceptions of them and how this has the potential to affect the data obtained. Informants will make judgements about what it is safe and acceptable to tell researchers. This may depend on the initial impression given and the personality of the researcher. This is vitally important in any social society that is hierarchical, as informants may state what they think the researcher wants to hear. This can be clarified by observing behaviour or by future data collected. Boyle (1994, p. 167) dislikes the term 'informant' because of its negative connotations and prefers the term 'participant', as it 'reflects the nature of the discourse and relationship between the researcher and the individuals who participate'. Members of the sample in classical anthropology used to be termed natives.

The use of emic and etic data

The researcher depends on participants within the field who may be interviewed to explore their point of view. Through an interview the researcher enters the participants' world of purpose, meaning and beliefs, seeing the culture through their eyes: this is the **emic perspective** and provides emic data. Emic data acknowledges that participants know better than the researcher. The **etic perspective** is obtained when the researcher attempts to make sense of that which is seen. It is therefore the researcher's interpretation of events and actions, but assumptions may be made about certain actions. These assumptions should be clarified during a later visit to the field. Boyle (1994) believes that it is essential to be clear whether the final analysis is from the emic or etic perspective.

When midwives undertake research in a maternity setting they tend to obtain an etic perspective. As they are familiar with the environment they could be considered as insiders and using the etic perspective enables them to make sense of what is happening from the outsider's viewpoint. In this way, midwives may become aware of assumptions they have accepted during their socialization into the profession. So midwives are helped to see themselves as others see them. This may be uncomfortable and can lead to change. Kirkham's (1987) work on information-giving demonstrated ways in which midwives' communication did not benefit clients and the mechanisms that clients used to gain information from midwives.

The end product is ethnography

Ethnography is not only a method of investigation, a research technique, but is also seen as the product of that investigation. Agar (1980) reiterates that ethnography can be the process of the investigation and the product, the written account.

COMPONENTS OF THE RESEARCH PROCESS

Ethnography is difficult to design as it may change as the study progresses. It is therefore difficult to be precise at the planning stage as to the exact research process. Seeking Ethics Committee approval can be problematic, as committee members may be more used to the quantitative paradigm and even if they are familiar with qualitative work this may not extend to ethnography. This may equally apply to health professionals. Kirkham (1987), discussing her proposed ethnographic research with consultant obstetricians, was asked where her questionnaire was. When planning an ethnographic study the following stages are usually considered:

◆ choice of topic
◆ prefieldwork preparation; location, sample and observer
◆ entering and collecting data in the field
◆ analysing and reporting data.

Choice of topic

The choice of topic usually derives from clinical practice. If it becomes apparent that the focus of the topic involves the exploration of a culture, then ethnography is the appropriate approach. Researchers should not, however, blindly enter the setting and collect data but have a specific focus or purpose.

Ideally you should not have, or you should set aside, any preconceived ideas about the culture to be studied.

Prefieldwork preparation

Location

Before 'entering the field' it must be decided where the research will take place. Ball (1993) considers selecting the location to be part of the sampling process, as the site will affect the participant sample and hence the data obtained. Selection of the setting should be made explicit. It may be a school, a hospital, a specific clinic, a classroom or a defined group. Selection may be based on the convenience of the setting, including accessibility for the researcher. It may be typical of a type of setting or even selected because of its atypical characteristics. Chamberlain (1996) chose a site where she was based for a midwifery refresher course.

Sample

The recruitment of participants is just as important in ethnography as it is in quantitative research. As ethnography takes place in a natural setting the sampling is therefore naturalistic. It is important to consider sampling prior to data collection but because it is also part of the data collection process it is considered under data collection.

Observer

The role of the researcher must be thought through carefully prior to entry to the study setting. The degree of personal interaction the researcher will engage in and the amount of information participants will be given about the study should be decided prior to data collection. Four kinds of researcher participation are classically seen in ethnography:

- ◆ complete participant
- ◆ participant-as-observer
- ◆ observer-as-participant
- ◆ complete observer.

Complete participant

In anthropological and classical ethnography the researcher usually enters the culture as a complete or full participant. This means that researchers adopt an insider role and their identity is not known to the group. This necessitates a certain degree of deception and access to the whole group may be limited because of the role adopted. Data collection becomes complicated because of the deception required and has included such devious means as hidden tape recorders. This could be considered unethical. The data collected is subject to bias and oversubjectivity but enables access to insider information that would otherwise be difficult to explore. The problem with this is that the individual personal culture of the researcher can interfere with the setting or the setting can impact so much on the researcher that they are criticized as **going native**. This means adopting the cultural identity of the society being studied. The researcher then has the very dubious role of being not only the researcher but also the researched.

Participant-as-observer

When adopting the participant-as-observer role the researcher enters the social life of those studied and sometimes assumes an insider role – often a snoop or shadow – but is known to be a researcher. This means that the researcher can request access to the whole group and is able to seek feedback and clarification on what is seen and its interpretation. The researcher must avoid feeling at home and this is more difficult for researchers who may be researching their own territory. To avoid going native the researcher must achieve a balance between integration with the group and professional separation.

Observer-as-participant

If the observer-as-participant role is adopted, the researcher's role is known to participants but there is only limited interaction with them. This role is typical of single-session data collections.

Complete observer

This is the opposite to the complete participant. The researcher observes interactions but does not contribute to the setting or society being studied. This can be problematic because the presence of the observer may influence and affect people's behaviour, depending on their understanding of why the observer is there. The researcher may be visual, behind a screen but known to be a witness, covert and hidden or totally removed and distanced from the social field. Use may be made of one-way mirrors or hidden video cameras. If the researcher's presence as a complete observer is known to participants, then the focus of the study may be overt or covert. For example Kirkham (1987) did not inform participants that the focus of her study was communication and therefore was able to observe the communication of midwives in a labour ward without them being aware that this was what was being observed. This brings to the fore the ethical nature of overt, covert and semicovert ethnography. It would now be considered unethical not to inform individuals that they were being observed.

The dilemma of the nonparticipant/participant dichotomy was focused for Hunt in the discussion of what she would wear in the labour ward (Hunt and Symonds 1995). She stated at the onset of her study of the labour ward culture that she was a midwife, and because of the intimate nature of childbirth needed to be seen as part of the culture, i.e. a professional, by the clients. However she decided not to wear uniform, as she might be seen as part of the care-giving force and some responsibility might be given to her, which would have conflicted with her research role of observer. Instead, she wore a white coat, because if she had worn ordinary clothes she might have been mistaken for a relative. However, she eventually saw this as a dishonest deception and took to wearing ordinary clothes as the study progressed (Hunt and Symonds 1995). Hunt set out to be an observer but had decided that she would participate 'in such a way as to produce a relaxed feeling about my presence' (Hunt and Symonds 1995, p. 47). Kirkham (1987) faced a similar dilemma; because she was an experienced midwife she made decisions about actions that she would participate in:

> I decided upon entering the field that I would not initiate as a midwife but that if asked I would continue a course of action already started if the person taking that action was to be absent for a short time. . . . I stressed that I would take no part in the care of 'my' patients during labour. (Kirkham 1987, p. 26)

Kirkham (1987) found balancing the nature of the study and professional responsibility to clients difficult. This was also experienced by Davies in her study of student midwives, when she thought that what was being taught in the classroom was not only incorrect but potentially dangerous and therefore refuted the incorrect statements and acted as a teacher and not a researcher (Davies 1996). It could also be said that at this point Davies was acting as a midwife with a responsibility according to the Midwives' rules and code of practice (UKCC 1998), to the clients that she was serving. Burden (1998), who looked at the role of curtain positioning within a maternity ward, felt that she had to drop the role of researcher in order to maintain the health of a woman and act as a midwife and therefore could no longer observe but had to participate in care. Through reflection she saw this as detrimental to the study, as data was seen as invalidated and lost. Reflection is therefore essential to identify any conflict between the roles of researcher and midwife. The researcher should be self-aware and reflect on how her/his professional responsibility can aid the data obtained rather than restrict it. Any conflict should be made explicit.

Danziger (1979), although an observer in the lives of pregnant women, also interacted:

> I developed quite positive, warm relationships with the women.... In my role as observer I found myself performing many functions for these women. I offered support and encouragement, especially during labour when one's physical and emotional endurance is often tested beyond imagined limits.... I massaged their backs, cushioned them in a pushing position, held the bedpan, fed them ice chips, wiped their foreheads, retrieved nurses for them. (Danziger 1979, p. 521–522)

The ethnographer therefore can participate in a range of interactions in a study. In most midwifery ethnographies the researcher is known to be a researcher at the commencement of the study but the full extent of their professional standing or aims may not be disclosed initially. The degree of participation can be seen as a continuum 'along which all practitioners and researchers dance' (Kirkham 1994, p. 391) and in reality this is what usually occurs.

Fieldwork-access

The researcher has to gain access to the research setting, i.e. the field. All access to the **fieldwork** must be negotiated, through **gate-keepers** who are in positions to facilitate access to the desired group of people. Gate-keepers need to be identified before the commencement of the study. Contact can be formal, via officials and people in authority, or informal, through personal contact and networks. Permission may not be immediately forthcoming, because of the gate-keeper's unfamiliarity with the ethnographic method. This may change with the increasing publication of ethnographies in midwifery. Ball (1993) suggests that access negotiated through formal channels may not be seen as access by those within the field. This is because permission granted by someone within the hierarchical structure of an organization has also to be negotiated with the person in authority within the fieldwork location. In health-care settings this may mean the sister on the ward or the professional, such as the midwife conducting the delivery, as well as the Head of Midwifery Services or even the General Manager. Hunt negotiated access via:

◆ the senior midwife
◆ the director of nursing services

- the unit general manager
- the chief area nursing officer
- three consultant obstetricians
- the committee chairman of the Division of Obstetrics and Gynaecology
- the senior midwife teacher
- the district general manager's secretary
- the Health Authority Ethics Committee (Hunt and Symonds 1995, p. 43).

This is a formidable list and it eventually took a total of 9 months to gain the required access. This should always be taken into account when planning any form of ethnographic study.

LeCompte and Preissle (1993) discuss how overidentification with the hierarchy may alienate the 'lower ranks'. Therefore, once access is negotiated the researcher should not maintain close links with gate-keepers, as this could alienate informants, which in the health service may be individual practitioners, health-care assistants or domestic staff.

Even after access to the field is gained, there need to be continuing local negotiations to gain entry to specific individuals. Davies (1996) continued negotiating access while in the field as each lecturer was personally introduced to her and consent obtained. Consent for access to individual situations involving clients also needs to be gained from the client, who could be seen to be in a vulnerable position. It is therefore extremely important that the researcher is not seen to be part of the 'system', as the client should feel able to decline without feeling that it would influence her care. It is also important that clients still see the researcher in a professional guise and not just as a voyeur, as this would also influence their agreement and participation. When negotiating access in order to observe one woman's labour, Kirkham was told: 'You can because you are a midwife, I wouldn't have a sociologist' (Kirkham 1987, p. 24).

As the quote above indicates, the status attributed to the researcher by the potential participant can influence the likelihood of her/him consenting to involvement in the study. While professional status can be helpful, other roles may be perceived as valid. For example, Hunt used the status of student to smooth introductions and gain local access. 'I used my standard introduction whenever I met anyone new to me. "Hello, I am a midwife studying part-time at the university, I am looking at. . ."' (Hunt and Symonds 1995, p. 46).

This sounds similar to negotiating the presence of midwifery, nursing or medical students within a health-care setting, and as such is a regular occurrence for midwives working within a teaching hospital. So midwives can be seen to have skills of negotiation, which they use every day within their practice, for ethnographic research.

Fieldwork

Immersion and language

Involvement in the culture is known as fieldwork and it involves researchers immersing themselves in the culture. Initially, the emphasis is on the field-work, immersion into the culture, rather than data collection. In anthropological ethnography, researchers would live within the culture they were exploring. This might necessitate learning the language and might take years. The use of language is not pertinent just for anthropological studies but also for health and social ethnography. To understand interaction it is necessary to under-stand the language, idiom or terminology of the society or group being studied. It could be considered that what people do is more important than what they say, but some researchers see mastery of language as crucial (LeCompte and Preissle 1993). This is just as important in the study of cultures such as the teenage culture or occupational groups such as mid-wives, where the familiarity with the setting may work in the researcher's favour. The researcher must be intellectually poised between familiarity and strangeness (Hammersley and Atkinson 1983). Hunt describes her position as being both 'on the outside and inside at the same time, and never really "at home"' (Hunt and Symonds 1995, p. 47). Davies reproduces an extract from her journal written during her fieldwork: 'I was familiar with the "jargon" of the occupational group I was studying. This, however, may be a double-edged sword as the ethnographer has to constantly remember to avoid "going native"' (Davies 1985, p. 225).

Timing and its difficulties

Once in the field, researchers usually spend time there on a continuous basis, with prolonged direct contact as seen in classical anthropology. This may necessitate whole weeks spent in the setting or a large selection of days. This is time-consuming and practitioners who are undertaking research in addition to practising their profession may find the ethnographic approach difficult because of the amount of time required. Some researchers only enter the field for specific times or events. Hunt (Hunt and Symonds 1995) arranged to observe handovers at shift changes and to be present at various times throughout the week, sometimes for a few hours and at other times for longer. Ball (1993) highlights the fact that the time of day is rarely mentioned in ethnographic reports but can be important, depending on the focus of the study. Schools have specific cycles within the year and so do hospitals. Junior doctor changeovers may affect the field when looking at the role of midwives within a hospital setting. Shift changeovers are important times. The differences between day, night and weekends may be vital as at these times the staffing roles may be quite different, with more being required of midwives in the absence of medical staff. Whatever time is selected by the researcher, it may be unsuitable because of the nature of midwifery and childbirth; for example, if a time is chosen in order to be present at a birth one may not be imminent. Chamberlain (1996) found the Special Care Baby Unit a difficult area to sample, in her study of clinical teaching of student midwives, because of the influx of seriously ill babies and the concomitantly large number of medical staff present whenever she decided to observe students. All these features show how the identification of study participants as data sources can be influenced by the research process.

Personal consequences

Fieldwork may involve or affect the researcher's family, especially if the researcher is a woman with children. O'Brien (1993) describes the visit of parents and brothers and sisters during her fieldwork. Sometimes, fieldwork is dangerous and this has led to the criticism of ethnographers as being thrill-seekers (Lee 1995). This is more obvious when looking at potentially violent subcultures such as drug abusers and youth gangs. Researchers need to be aware of potential health problems, especially if the fieldwork takes place overseas. Female researchers may face sexual harassment and are aware of a greater pressure than male fieldworkers to have sexual relations within the field (Bell et al 1993).

Collection of data

The principal tool for data collection in ethnographic studies is the researcher. This does not preclude the use of other tools, such as observation and interviews (Chamberlain 1996), but these are very confining. LeCompte and Preissle (1993) suggest that the sources and types of data collection within ethnographic research are wide and dependent on the creativity and energy of the researcher. This data can be divided into interactive and non-interactive (Pelto and Pelto 1978). Interactive data requires the researcher to interact with the participants, which may lead to reactions that affect the data. Noninteractive data requires no interaction with participants by the researcher.

Noninteractive data

Such data may consist of descriptions about the physical state of the site and how it is laid out. Hunt (Hunt and Symonds 1995) describes how the chairs were laid out in the office of a labour ward. It may include nonparticipant observation. Some researchers may be specific with regard to their observations and record how people use space; this is called **proxemics**.

Archival material can be used. In health-care settings this may mean clients' medical notes or care plans, protocols and procedure documents. Burden (1998) used notes and care charts to obtain details of type of delivery, method of feeding and other factors considered to be relevant to her study on the use of curtain positioning within a maternity ward. This was to 'build a picture of the possible extenuating factors that could influence the way in which women acted within the ward environment' (Burden 1998, p. 18). Photographs may also be useful (Machin and Scammell 1997).

Initial observations may be unfocused and Chamberlain (1996) found that observation was not easy despite the fact that she was a midwife: 'It took a little time for me to realize that observing someone's condition required a different set of skills from that needed for the observation of an interaction' (Chamberlain 1996, p. 113).

Interactive data

This involves interacting with participants and involves records of conversations and interviews. Tape recorders may be used for formal interviews. Selecting appropriate people within the setting to observe or interview is vital for the study and they must be chosen with care (Hammersley and Atkinson 1983). This does not mean that the key informant is seen as an authority within the field; they may be a health-care assistant or a cleaner. It is also important to acknowledge that some people may want to be interviewed because they feel that they have something important to say because they are following their own agendas. This was found by Hunt, as staff midwives were anxious to join in a group discussion and to tell of all the 'stresses and negative features of being a midwife' (Hunt and Symonds 1995, p. 123). Sometimes it is obvious who is a key informant.

Interviews

Interviews may occur throughout the period of data collection and can be used as a thermometer that gauges the validity of the analysis. Interviews will be unstructured but directed and focused and the researcher may compile a list of areas to cover. The reliability of data collected by interviews can be checked by using other methods, such as observation.

Field notes

Field notes are often taken during the study and immediately on leaving the field. This necessitates the use of a notebook during observations or immediately afterwards. Some researchers consider a clipboard or a notebook as 'off-putting' for participants, whereas others may see it as an overt tool of their trade, which acknowledges their position as researcher rather than midwife. Kirkham (1987) saw note-taking as a part of the culture being studied. Hunt (Hunt and Symonds 1995) used a Dictaphone in a store cupboard or a toilet in order to record key phrases and other prompts.

What to record in field notes can be a problem and Hunt (Hunt and Symonds 1995) used Spradley's (1980) checklist, which can be seen as a useful guide, especially for the novice ethnographer and is shown in Box 7.2.

Box 7.2 An example of what can be recorded in field notes

◆ Space: physical places
◆ Actors: people involved
◆ Activity: sets of related acts that people do
◆ Objects: the physical things that are present
◆ Acts: single actions that people do
◆ Event: a set of related activities that people carry out
◆ Time: the sequencing that takes place over time
◆ Goals: things people are trying to accomplish
◆ Feelings: emotions felt and expressed

Data analysis and reporting

Ethnographic analysis involves the search for patterns in the data and ideas which help explain the existence of the patterns (Boyle 1994). Data analysis tends to be an ongoing process. Boyle (1994) divides the analysis of ethnographic data into three areas:

◆ cognitive ethnographies (ethnoscience)
◆ content analysis
◆ text/descriptive analysis.

Cognitive ethnographies

This is a complex form of analysis and is usually performed by anthropologists and social scientists, especially those undertaking systematic ethnography. It involves the development of folk taxonomies, which are a description of how people connect specific concepts together and could be seen as similar to concept mapping. Cultural themes may be developed and these may be divided into major and minor.

Content analysis

This is a term which is used to cover a number of techniques which make inferences from textual data. It can be used with any form of text and so can be used for observational data, as well as transcripts of interviews. Silverman (1993) sees **content analysis** as quantitative and therefore dismisses it as a qualitative form of textual analysis. There are two main types:

◆ manifest content analysis
◆ latent content analysis.

These involve categorizing words or phrases with a conceptual label that describes it. A computer can then be used to count how many times a particular word or phrase appears. When latent content analysis is used the researcher goes beyond what is said or written and attempts to uncover meaning.

Descriptive analysis

This is a traditional approach to analysing ethnographic data. The analysis commences early in the study and continues throughout. As the ethnographer develops ideas they are tested against observations and vice versa. There is a 'back and forth' process of data collection and analysis, involving switching from emic to etic perspectives and testing them against each other. It is here that confusion occurs with the grounded theory form of analysing data. Other researchers describe it as decontextualizing and recontextualizing text data (Boyle 1994). Chamberlain (1996, 1997), in her study of clinical teaching, used the grounded theory approach of constant comparative analysis for the analysis of data collected via ethnography.

In analysing documents Hammersley and Atkinson (1983, p. 142–143) encourage the posing of questions such as:

◆ How are the documents written?
◆ How are they read?
◆ Who writes them?
◆ Who reads them?
◆ For what purposes?
◆ On what occasions?
◆ With what outcomes?
◆ What is recorded?
◆ What is omitted?
◆ What is taken for granted?

◆ What does the writer seem to take for granted about the reader?

◆ What do readers need to know to make sense of them?

Ethnographic reports

The list above is also a good guide for what to write in the report of an ethnographic study. Ethnographies normally take the form of books with an easy-to-read narrative style, as condensing data may lose its meaning. This may be one reason why less qualitative studies are published in midwifery or medical journals as short articles. They are normally written in the first person, in keeping with the recognized subjectivity of the data, which is an anathema in quantitative approaches, which attempt to give the illusion of objectivity.

CONCLUSION

Having explored the process of ethnographic research you can see that the boundaries of ethnography are not precise, as they overlap with other qualitative approaches. The ethnographer sets out on an unknown voyage and as such this journey has been likened to a combination of *Star Trek* and *Mission Impossible* (Ball 1993). The researcher may not be bold, s/he may set out in fear and trepidation unprotected by a distinct research protocol or a sheaf of questionnaires. However, ethnography can allow pregnancy, parenthood, childbirth and many other social states to be seen from a differing perspective and as such has a lot to offer midwives and the midwifery profession.

CHAPTER SUMMARY

This chapter has highlighted that:

Ethnography provides the means by which a culture can be explored.

◆ The sample originates from within the culture.

◆ The researcher becomes immersed in the culture.

◆ Data are collected using participant or nonparticipant observation, description of the setting, and archival material.

◆ Field notes are recorded.

◆ Approaches to analysis differ but focus on interpreting and understanding behaviour and interactions within the culture. This is achieved from the emic and etic perspective.

Ethnography can be the process of the investigation and the product, which is the written account.

REFERENCES

Agar M 1980 The professional stranger: an informal introduction to ethnography. Academic Press, New York

Ball S J 1993 Self-doubt and soft data: social and technical trajectories in ethnographic fieldwork. In: Hammersley M (ed) Educational research, current issues, vol 1, Paul Chapman, London, ch 3, p 32–48

Bell D, Caplan P, Karim W J (ed) 1993 Gendered fields, women, men and ethnography. Routledge, London

Boas F 1924 The methods of ethnology. American Anthropologist 22: 311–321

Boyle 1994 Styles of ethnography. In: Morse J M (ed) Critical issues in qualitative research methods. Sage Publications, Thousand Oaks, ch 9, p 159–186

Burden B 1998 Privacy or help? The use of curtain positioning strategies within the maternity ward environment as a means of achieving and maintaining privacy, or as a form of signalling to peers and professionals in an attempt to seek information or support. Journal of Advanced Nursing 27(1): 15–23

Chamberlain M 1996 The clinical education of student midwives. In: Robinson S, Thompson A (ed) Midwives, research and childbirth, vol 4. Chapman & Hall, London, ch 6, p 108–132

Chamberlain M 1997 Challenges of clinical learning for student midwives. Midwifery 13(2): 85–91

Danziger S K 1979 On doctor watching: field work in medical settings. Urban Life 17(4): 513–532

Davies L 1985 Ethnography and status: focusing on gender in educational research. In: Burgess R (ed) Field methods in the study of education, vol 1. Falmer Press, Lewes, ch 4, p 79–96

Davies R 1996 'Practitioners in their own right': an ethnographic study of the perceptions of student midwives. In: Robinson S, Thompson A (ed) Midwives, research and childbirth, vol 4. Chapman & Hall, London, ch 5, p 85–108

Hammersley M, Atkinson P 1983 Ethnography: principles in practice, vol 1. Tavistock, London

Hunt S, Symonds A 1995 The social meaning of midwifery. Macmillan, Basingstoke

Jacobson D 1991 Reading ethnography. State University of New York Press, Albany, NY

Jordan B 1980 Birth in four cultures. Eden Press, Montreal, Quebec

Kirkham M 1987 Basic supportive care in labour: interaction with and around women in labour. PhD thesis, University of Manchester

Kirkham M 1994 Using research skills in midwifery practice. British Journal of Midwifery 2(8): 390–392

LeCompte M D, Preissle J 1993 Ethnography and qualitative design in educational research, 2nd edn. Academic Press, London

Lee R M 1995 Dangerous fieldwork. Qualitative research methods, vol 34. Sage Publications, London

Leininger M M 1985 Ethnography and ethnonursing: models and modes of qualitative data analysis. In: Leininger M M (ed) Qualitative research methods in nursing. WB Saunders, Philadelphia, PA, ch 3, p 33–71

Lipson J 1991 The use of self in ethnographic research. In: Morse J (ed) Qualitative nursing research: a contemporary dialogue. Sage Publications, London, ch 5, p 73–90

Machin D, Scamell M 1997 The experience of labour: using ethnography to explore the irresistible nature of the bio-medical metaphor during labour. Midwifery 13(2): 78–84

Mead M 1929 Coming of age in Samoa. New American Library, New York

Morse J, Field P A 1996 Nursing research: the application of qualitative approaches, 2nd edn. Chapman & Hall, London

Muecke M 1994 On the evaluation of ethnographies. In: Morse J M (ed) Critical issues in qualitative research methods. Sage Publications, Thousand Oaks, CA, ch 10, p 187–210

O'Brien O 1993 Sisters, parents, neighbours, friends: Reflections on fieldwork in North Catalonia (France). In: Bell D, Caplan P, Karim W J (ed) Gendered fields, vol 1. Routledge, London, ch 13, p 234–248

Pelto P J, Pelto G H 1978 Anthropological research: the structure of inquiry, 2nd edn. Cambridge University Press, Cambridge

Silverman D 1993 Interpreting qualitative data. Sage Publications, London

Spradley J P 1980 Participant observation. Holt, Rinehart, & Winston, New York

Symonds A, Hunt S 1996 The midwife and society: perspectives, policies and practice, vol 1. Macmillan, Basingstoke

UKCC 1998 Midwives' rules and code of practice. UKCC, London

Werner O, Schoepfle G M 1987 Systematic fieldwork, vol 2. Sage Publications, Newbury Park, CA

8

Phenomenology

Ann Robinson

INTRODUCTION

Phenomenology is an approach used within qualitative research that permits the researcher to delve into and gain an understanding of otherwise poorly understood **phenomena**. The concept of phenomenology may be difficult to understand. The aim of this chapter is to remove some of the mystique surrounding this approach and to place it in a context that may be of use to midwives exploring the art of qualitative research. Midwives undertaking a phenomenological study will be required to explain the process and its background to justify their approach in a report or dissertation. To help midwives achieve this, phenomenology has been considered from a historical perspective as well as discussing its interpretation by contemporary scholars. Issues relating to the approach, such as suitable methods of data collection, sampling and data analysis, have been focused upon from a phenomenological perspective, as have the complexities of ensuring **trustworthiness**.

ORIGINS

Phenomenology grew out of a need to understand the effects of experience on individuals (Clarke and Wheeler 1992, Talbot 1995). It derives from Greek *phainomenon*, meaning 'appearance' and *logos*, meaning 'reason' (Walters 1995) and refers to 'the study of everyday life as it is actually lived and experienced' (Bottorff 1990, p. 202) or, as described by Edmund Husserl (1967, p. 452), an 'essential science of Non-realities'.

It is useful to place phenomenology in a historical perspective. There are several differing interpretations that underlie phenomenology (Omery 1983, Stewart and Mickunas 1990, Reed 1994), which are now well appreciated (Paley 1998). Phenomenology may be traced to the 18th century, to its philosophical ancestors (Baker et al 1992, Jasper 1994) and scholars of transcendental, existentialist and hermeneutic philosophy such as Husserl and Heidegger (Reed 1994). 'Existentialist' means existence through experience rather than reason, while 'hermeneutic' relates to interpretation (Walters, 1995) and originates from the Greek word *hermeneia* (Annells 1996). 'Transcendental' refers to the vision of Husserl, a great pioneer in the quest for the acceptance of phenomenology and a believer that it was 'a science of the cognition of essences rather than of matters of fact' (Annells 1996, p. 706).

Herbert Spiegelberg (1965) placed phenomenology on to its historical pathway by dividing its development into stages or parts, for example the early stage, German stage and French stage. Each stage may be exemplified by specific noteworthy exponents of phenomenology. Immanuel Kant is reputed as being the first to use the word 'phenomenology', in 1786, in an attempt to illustrate the importance of focusing on the appearance of phenomena or things (Cohen 1987). According to Spiegelberg (1965), Franz Brentano (1838–1917) and Carl Stumpf (1848–1936) were at an early stage particularly inspirational and focused on what were to become key phenomenological concepts such as inner perception and intentionality. Cohen (1987, p. 32) describes inner perception as us having an 'awareness of our own psychic phenomena' and intentionality as relating to the idea 'that everything that we consider to be psychical refers to an object'.

Edmond Husserl (1859–1938), a German philosopher and lecturer, and an apostle of Brentano and Stumpf, is generally considered to be founder of the phenomenological movement (Stewart and Mickunas 1990) and of key importance in the classification of transcendental phenomenology (Annells 1996). Husserl was excited by the development of the natural sciences in the late 19th century (Omery 1983) and aspired to provide philosophy with the same interpretation and recognition as that attributed to the rigorous sciences (Walters 1995), very much 'in the same way that nonhuman phenomena are studied, from a detached, rather than emotionally involved stance' (Reed 1994, p. 337). Husserl held a belief that, in order to obtain real understanding of any phenomena (experience or happening), one must become in touch with one's own conscious state (Husserl 1967) and able to interpret the basis of experience and therefore the essence of that experience (Spiegelberg 1965). While interpreting the essence of an experience, Husserl proposed the need to consider reduction. This process of reduction or bracketing focuses on the need to suspend our beliefs (Spiegelberg 1965) in order to interpret the true meaning of a phenomenon.

According to Cohen (1987, p. 32), Husserl felt that phenomenology was 'the universal foundation of philosophy and science' and today, Husserl's term *Lebenswelt*, **lived experience**, is synonymous with phenomenology (Jasper 1994), as is **intersubjectivity**, the existence of a belief that a shared experience can exist (Husserl 1967, Cohen 1987).

Martin Heidegger (1889–1976), also a German philosopher and successor to Husserl at Freiberg University (1929–1945), was a great influence on other phenomenologists, in particular, Gabriel Marcel (1889–1973), the renowned French philosopher, writer Jean-Paul Sartre (1905–1980) and Maurice Merleau-Ponty (1908–1961); (Cohen 1987, Jasper 1994). Heidegger is renowned for concentrating on another branch of phenomenology, that of hermeneutic phenomenology and a belief in *dasein* (Annells 1996). This German word translates as 'being-in-the-world' (Reed 1994), meaning that a person cannot be understood outside the context of their environment or world (Walters 1995). In taking this translation a stage further, Reed (1994) described three differing elements: 'attunement or mood', 'discourse or articulation', which relates things to their function and thirdly, organizing the environment to achieve a goal (Reed 1994, p. 337–338).

It is hard not to consider Heidegger without focusing on his commitment to Nazism during the late 1930s and 1940s (Holmes 1996). According to Cohen (1987, p. 33) 'Heidegger's Nazi involvement ended his activism as well as his trust in human beings and the power of subjectivity' and perhaps ultimately ended the intensity of this German phase within the development of phenomenology. It is possible that Heidegger's association with Nazism may have affected some individuals' perceptions of phenomenology.

Following the Second World War phenomenology firmly took its resting place in France (Cohen 1987) and continued to be debated and developed. Jean-Paul Sartre and Maurice Merleau-Ponty, both literary experts, to name but two (Spiegelberg 1965), became infamous practitioners. Key concepts at this time focused on the belief that how individuals act or behave is based on their awareness and perception of the phenomenon (Streubert and Carpenter 1999).

PURPOSE

Midwives are beginning to gain experience in the use of phenomenology (Bottorff 1990, Reed 1994, Beck 1994, Halldorsdottir and Karlsdottir 1996). This approach provides midwives with a framework in which to explore the needs and experiences of women encountering the childbearing process, at a depth often not previously sought. It brings feelings and experiences to life, enabling others to catch a glimpse of the otherwise unknown. It calls for the participant to interpret an experience and for the researcher to interpret that interpretation (Burns and Grove 1993). Later in the chapter it will be shown that midwives have a number of skills that can help them fulfil the purposes of phenomenological enquiry and these, Halldorsdottir and Karlsdottir (1996) believe, prevent the true spirit of the experience from being lost during the process of interpretation.

The knowledge and understanding gained by adopting a phenomenological perspective can help midwives to fulfil the definition of a midwife, to be 'with woman' (Donnison 1988, p. 11) and facilitate improvements in practice. Seeking knowledge in an attempt to facilitate the needs of childbearing women also corresponds to the French translation of midwife, *sage-femme*, meaning 'wise woman' (Gelis 1991, p. 105).

Incorporated within the philosophy of midwifery is the provision of individualized care based on the physical, social, psychological, emotional, spiritual and educational needs of women. Care therefore emphasizes the whole person rather than one particular element. Phenomenology attempts to understand all aspects of a phenomenon in preference to concentrating on a specific concept, and therefore has a reverence for caring for the whole that is admirably suited to midwifery.

CHARACTERISTICS OF THE APPROACH

A multiplicity of definitions and interpretations of phenomenology are familiar to contemporary scholars. In spite of phenomenology's plethora of historical interpretation, many still question whether phenomenology is a research approach and confuse many of its elements with qualitative research in general. Indeed, the following definition relating to qualitative research may well apply to phenomenology: 'The exploration of little-known phenomena that are not easily qualified or categorized using inductive reasoning to develop generalizations or theories from specific observations or interviews' (Talbot 1995, p. 658).

Phenomenology appreciates that the complexity of life's experiences deserves more than a cursory, superficial glance. It enables depth to be viewed within the context of those experiencing the phenomenon and is reputed to enable otherwise complex experiences to come alive and be understood. This has been described as a 'science whose purpose is to describe particular phenomena, or the appearance of things, as lived experience' (Streubert and Carpenter 1999, p. 43).

Oiler (1982) clearly describes phenomenology as an approach, a method and a philosophy, while Omery (1983, p. 50), in comprehensively analysing the use of phenomenology in nursing, describes phenomenology as being 'an inductive, descriptive research method'. The aim is to explore or investigate the phenomenon and describe it in detail as it occurs in real life. This includes consideration of how individuals and the phenomenon interact.

Morse (1992, p. 91), in attempting to capture the essence of phenomenology, perceives that 'it is the uniqueness of living that is vital, that makes our life ours, and that is sought in phenomenological expression'. Similarly, Powers and Knapp (1995, p. 123) describe phenomenology as being 'a way of thinking about what life experiences are like for people'.

Oiler (1982), in an attempt to emphasize the many interpretations of phenomenology, identified four characteristics or features, which are listed in Box 8.1.

Box 8.1 Characteristics of phenomenology (Oiler 1982)

◆ **Phenomena:** this refers to the significant appearance of objects and events.

◆ **Reality:** Oiler (1982, p. 178–179) describes this as being 'subjective and perspectival'. This means that reality relies heavily on the interpretation of an appearance and is coloured by individuality and thus may be arbitrary.

◆ **Subjectivity:** meaning that the world becomes real by being in touch with it, and therefore

◆ **Truth** finally develops from individual expression.

Several interpretations are frequently tested by contemporary scholars, for example the van Kaam method, the Giorgi method and the Colaizzi method (Omery 1983). All call for experiences to be recalled and described in order that a true understanding is ascertained. Before these interpretations are considered, it is useful to focus upon some common threads. Herbert Spiegelberg (1965) acknowledges that phenomenological inquiry is made up of a number of components, all of which are important and can be followed in sequential order. It is not however essential to include all components in a study (Box 8.2).

Suspending one's memory, experience or even beliefs to avoid preconceived

---

Box 8.2 Classification of phenomenology (Omery 1983)

◆ **Descriptive phenomenology** explores, describes and analyses phenomena

◆ **Phenomenology of the essences** is viewing and exploring the phenomena for typical structures or 'essentials' and for the relationship between structures

◆ **Phenomenology of appearances** is observing the phenomena from different perspectives to achieve clarity

◆ **Constitutive phenomenology** is the exploration of the ways in which phenomena are formed or shaped in the mind of the individuals

◆ **Reductive phenomenology** is putting to one side your own beliefs to view the phenomena from the perspective of participants ... 'bracketing'

◆ **Hermeneutic phenomenology** is uncovering the covert meaning of the phenomena.

---

expectations sounds almost impossible to achieve. In practice, bracketing is facilitated by:

◆ selecting a research area unfamiliar to yourself
◆ postponing a review of the literature until all the data has been obtained (Oiler 1982, Streubert and Carpenter 1999)
◆ refraining from entering into any form of discussion with colleagues with regards to data collected (very important from a confidentiality perspective).

It is important to have a clear understanding of the philosophical under-pinnings of phenomenology, as well as a perspective on the multiplicity of definitions and interpretations of phenomenology by contemporary scholars. This comprehension facilitates the planning and implementation of the research study.

COMPONENTS OF THE PHENOMENOLOGICAL PROCESS

Sampling

Since many phenomenological studies necessitate the use of in-depth inter-views (Lundgren and Dahlberg 1998, Berg and Dahlberg 1998), the sample size may be small and selective. Size does not, however, reflect the amount of data available or the depth of investigation that is possible. Morse and Field

(1996) highlight that random sampling is inappropriate in qualitative research and emphasize the importance of collecting rich experiential data. Phenomenology is well suited to **purposeful sampling** (Streubert and Carpenter 1999). This type of sampling permits the selection of interviewees whose qualities or experiences permit an understanding of the phenomenon in question and are therefore invaluable. Patton (1990) suggests that this is the strength of purposeful sampling. One form of purposeful sampling is **snowball** or chain referral. This is appropriate when an experience is known to be rare, for example giving birth to an infant who is subsequently found to have phenylketonuria. This involves one mother with an affected child recommending other mothers with a similarly affected child who might be willing to participate in the study.

Data collection

In order to explore the 'lived experience', several methods of data collection may be contemplated. Diaries are a written record of events experienced by participants that are made available to researchers for analysis (Burns and Grove 1993). They have been successfully used in nursing research (Richardson 1994). For example, Oleske et al (1990) used diaries in order to gain insight into the lives of cancer patients. A diary commenced following the birth of a baby may provide the intimacy and confidentiality in which to describe personal experiences. A diary may enable participants to confide at once, instead of relying on memory later on (Roughman and Haggerty 1972). Robson (1993) and Richardson (1994), however, warn that diaries can prove problematic, since the participant is heavily depended upon. Problems relating to recruitment and the acquisition of reduced-quality data associated with diaries appear to act as common obstacles to their use.

The integration of research approaches (triangulation) could be considered in order to minimize method imperfections and obtain an enactment of the phenomenon being studied. According to DePoy and Gitlin (1994, p. 150), triangulation in naturalistic research is entitled 'a multistrategy approach', the purpose of which is to attempt to explore all avenues and dimensions. Winter (1989) believes that three different methods should be used so that comparisons can be made and any limitations associated with a method overcome. Questionnaires followed by semistructured interviews may, for example, provide 'completeness' (DePoy and Gitlin 1994, p. 150), a term used to reflect a holistic picture of the differing aspects to a study. Participants may feel happier and less inhibited by initially responding on paper rather than face to face. The absence of a researcher would also protect against bias due to the researcher's reactions or responses (Polit and Hungler 1997). Another advantage of using questionnaires prior to interviewing is that participants have the opportunity to consider their responses. For further discussion regarding the benefits and complexities of triangulation, you can refer to Chapter 9.

The interview

Recent evidence exists to reflect the popularity among phenomenologists of selecting 'the interview' as a method of data collection (Bottorff 1990, Beck 1994, Reed 1994, Halldorsdottir and Karlsdottir 1996, Lundgren and Dahlberg 1998, Berg and Dahlberg 1998). Phenomenologists often favour the intimacy that in-depth interviewing can create in an attempt to understand little known phenomena. Interviewing is a popular and widely used method of data collection (Fielding 1994). The interview may facilitate a process of exploration and offer a sense of freedom, enabling participants to steer the interview from their personal perspective. Interviews may at times be led by the interviewer, while at other times the interviews may be steered by the participant's replies into areas previously not considered. The use of open-ended, clarifying questions is particularly helpful (Streubert and Carpenter 1999). They necessitate considerable freedom, enabling participants to speak openly and candidly about experiences personal to themselves. This freedom often constitutes something of 'an adventure' (Rose 1994, p. 25).

The relationship midwives have with the women they care for may facilitate the collection of data. Being 'with woman' highlights the midwife's close relationship with the client and emphasizes the midwife's role as a woman's advocate. Empathy, intimacy and a oneness with the woman are implicit within this relationship. Trust is also crucial to the relationship, as Lundgren and Dahlberg (1998) revealed in a study of women's experiences of pain in childbirth. These are all essential characteristics of the phenomenological relationship. Midwives therefore possess qualities that promote a unique closeness and a comfortable, safe, relaxed, environment in which women feel safe to reveal their innermost feelings, anxieties and experiences. This can be enhanced by the provision of privacy and confidentiality.

Interviewing involves two people being able to communicate with each other and midwives also possess the communication skills necessary for an approach that is both intimate and searching. Gelis (1991), in an exploration of the historical role of the midwife, described the 18th century midwife as someone who was 'reassuring... she knew how to make the right gestures; she said words of comfort and delivered' (Gelis 1991, p. 105). In this description Gelis has emphasized the importance of communication as well as knowledge, which are equally important today. Skills associated with listening and seeking meaning are particularly relevant. Communication contributes towards creating the environment which is imperative if the conversation is to flow naturally and participants are to remain relaxed, unreserved and uninhibited (Garrett, 1982). If you use a tape recorder to record these conversations it is important to ensure that it records consistently and clearly. It can also be helpful to take a notebook with you because as soon as the tape recorder is switched off participants frequently provide you with rich data.

Analysing the data

Phenomenologists seek to ensure that data analysis enables the meaning of the phenomenon to be understood while preserving the individuality of each participant's experience (Banonis 1989). The meaning of the phenomenon comes gradually and as a result of careful and repeated listening, reading and reflecting. You will need to listen to the recordings several times to become familiar with the responses. Pay special attention to participants' tone of voice, hesitations, sighs and laughter. These are all part of the phenomenon in question. If possible, it is best to personally transcribe the recordings. This process, however slow, does permit this familiarity to grow and allows the researcher to become further immersed in the data.

Several phenomenological interpretations exist and the features of those of van Kaam (1959), Giorgi (1970, 1985) and Colaizzi (1978) are outlined in Box 8.3.

These interpretations have common features. From an analysis perspective, they begin with the transcribing of data, and this is coded into themes. Key words that signify the identification of themes are usually clear and easily noticed. Lundgren and Dahlberg (1998, p. 106) call these 'meaning units'. Similar themes are incorporated to form categories and, finally, attributes of the phenomenon are highlighted (Jasper 1994). Contemporary scholars often base their phenomenological analysis on the interpretations or approaches shown above (Clarke and Wheeler 1992, Beck 1994, Robinson 1995, Lundgren and Dahlberg 1998). Colaizzi (1978) highlights a user-friendly guide to analysis, one that can be used by both novice and experienced researchers. It is a step-by-step guide, leading to a clear description of the phenomenon in question (Robinson 1995). Which approach you adopt will, however, depend on the phenomenon that is being explored and knowledge gained from the literature (Holloway and Wheeler 1996). Other approaches to data analysis are also available and researchers are not confined to the three presented in this chapter.

Mills (1994) believes that it is best to begin analysing the data as soon as the initial data has been collected, since this will act as a guide to further data collection. Data analysis is then ongoing. Streubert and Carpenter (1999), however, suggest that all the data you need can be collected and then analysed.

Midwife researchers might favour the freedom phenomenology provides in exploring the depth of a lived phenomenon pertaining to the childbearing continuum (Bottorff 1990, Beck 1994, Halldorsdottir and Karlsdottir 1996).

Box 8.3 Methods of phenomenological interpretation

Adrian L. van Kaam (1959)

◆ Establish a core of common experiences.

◆ Enable participants to freely express themselves. Participants may use a variety of ways to do this and, although this breadth may ultimately not be required, bias due to the researcher's philosophy may be avoided.

◆ Reduction and elimination. This involves recognizing and naming the important aspects of the phenomenon, thus reducing the data and eliminating what is irrelevant to the study.

◆ All commonalities are tentatively collected together in clusters and labelled.

◆ The final identification of the descriptive constituents. Each relevant constituent or component is identified to reveal the essential structure of the phenomenon.

Giorgi (1970, 1985)

◆ Preliminary overview of the phenomenon following an interview with a participant.

◆ Further reading of the description of this phenomenon.

◆ Separate parts of the description are identified following further consideration.

◆ Individual parts are considered alone and in relation to each other.

◆ The identified parts are reflected upon. The meaning is then transformed 'into the language or concepts of the science' (Omery 1983, p. 52).

◆ A description is then released, which is open to others for analysis.

Colaizzi (1978)

◆ Collection of data from participants.

◆ Examination of interview transcripts.

◆ Extraction of phrases directly related to the phenomenon.

◆ Consideration of the meaning of these phrases.

◆ Extraction of themes from the interpretation of the phrases.

◆ The themes then become a description of the phenomenon.

◆ Returning to the participants with the results to check for trustworthiness.

Beck (1994), selecting Colaizzi's (1978) phenomenological interpretation, explored women's thoughts and feelings during labour and delivery. Beck's findings highlight many implications for midwifery practice, especially the need to repeat information and to check understanding at this unique and sensitive time. Bottorff (1990), keen to understand why mothers choose and continue to breastfeed, used phenomenology successfully to describe feelings such as commitment and the need to give.

Literature review

Do remember the importance of encountering phenomena from as fresh a perspective as possible. To do this you need to 'bracket' or suspend your own beliefs (Spiegelberg 1965) so that you can interpret the true meaning of phenomena. It is, however, impossible to eradicate all previous knowledge and experiences. One recommendation is to focus on the literature review towards the end of the study, thereby minimizing data contamination. Apart from critically analysing literature relating to the phenomenon being explored, it is also advantageous to analyse phenomenological literature, both historical and contemporary. This provides an insight and comparison with regard to the numerous interpretations.

Trustworthiness

Trustworthiness is an essential component of qualitative research. Findings should reflect the reality of the experience. Trustworthiness therefore refers to the accuracy and honesty of the data (Oiler 1982). This trustworthiness or credibility can be identified by providing participants with the opportunity to review the researcher's interpretation of the data (Koch 1994, Guba and Lincoln 1989). Colaizzi (1978) suggests that participants should be presented with a description of the phenomenon and asked to verify the researcher's interpretations. Any new data obtained from participants can then be incorporated into the final description. Benner (1994), however, supports the use of a counselling approach to data collection – for example, the use of repetition and reflection: 'is that what you mean…?' This acts as an ongoing process and prevents the possibility of a 'second account' occurring. Beck (1994) checked each participant's understanding on completion of an interview. In this way the first and only account of the given phenomenon was obtained and participant confidentiality was maintained.

Team analysis provides the investigator with an opportunity to gain many interpretations of the data and therefore prevent bias. This may be questionable, since it would involve multiple data translation by individuals not closely involved with participants, the research process, or indeed the phenomenon being studied. From a confidentiality perspective, participants would need to consent to their responses being analysed by several people.

Bracketing contributes to trustworthiness by helping researchers ensure that their beliefs do not influence the collection of data and its analysis. In this way, biased results can be avoided and a reliable description of a given phenomenon provided (Beck 1994).

When considering the importance of trustworthiness, dependability, transferability and confirmability (Guba and Lincoln 1989) are also issues that need to be addressed. In order to ensure a qualitative study's dependability, another researcher would need to travel the same pathway, resulting in similar findings (Talbot 1995). This means that the original researcher must provide what Lincoln and Guba (1985) call an 'audit trail', which makes explicit each step of the research process. Transferability refers to whether the findings of a study can be applied to other settings that are similar. When data can be linked to the participants from whom it was derived it is said to have confirmability (Guba and Lincoln 1989). This applies to the findings of the study, interpretations and conclusions. A study that has been demonstrated to be credible, transferable and dependable can also be said to be confirmable (Lincoln and Guba 1985).

ETHICAL CONSIDERATIONS

Any research planning should culminate in the acquisition of ethical approval. Ethics in research can be considered to be the degree to which the research conforms to moral standards, including issues related to professional, legal and social accountability. Phenomenological enquiry is largely dependent on the participation of carefully selected individuals, in order that a particular phenomenon may be truly visualized. As with all research participants, harm and exploitation must be avoided (Polit and Hungler 1997) and therefore beneficence needs careful consideration. In order to prevent psychological damage being inflicted on participants, questions must be carefully selected and asked in a sensitive and caring manner. Debriefing sessions immediately following interviews may be incorporated, allowing the interviewees time to reflect and ask questions.

With regard to freedom from exploitation, clear and concise information must be given to participants at all stages of the research process and all guidelines must be adhered to. Informed consent is essential, demonstrating that the participant's decision to partake was optional, having received accurate, clear and detailed information.

The following must always be emphasized:

◆ participants have the right to choose not to participate
◆ participants may terminate their participation at any point
◆ participants should be encouraged to ask for explanations at any stage.

Phenomenological enquiry is often personal and intimate and the maintenance of privacy is therefore paramount (Morse and Field 1996). It is important to guarantee that:

◆ the research is not too intrusive
◆ all data is maintained securely
◆ pseudonyms are used throughout to protect identity.

Ethical approval must be sought from the appropriate Ethics Committee before proceeding with the study. Ethics Committees have differing expectations. It is advantageous to consult either the chairman of the Ethical Committee or the individual nursing/midwifery representative when planning the study. It may also be appropriate to approach relevant hospital managers for their authorization, and indeed support.

CONCLUSION

Phenomenology seeks to explore the 'lived' experience of individuals and is therefore an appropriate approach for midwives to adopt in order to gain women's perspectives of the childbirth process, maternity services and issues related to their health care. Midwives have many skills that can contribute to the successful undertaking of phenomenological research; however, these same skills are of value to other research approaches and to the modification of research methods to meet the specific needs of women. In the next chapter, alternative approaches to research will be considered.

CHAPTER SUMMARY

This chapter has highlighted that:

◆ Phenomenology is derived from philosophy and focuses on the lived experience of individuals.

◆ It involves bracketing or suspension of your own beliefs.

◆ A purposive sample is collected.

◆ Data are collected using in-depth interviews and diaries.

◆ Data analysis will depend on the phenomenological interpretation adopted but includes:
  – examination of transcripts
  – identifying phrases related to the phenomenon and their meaning
  – establishing common themes
  – providing a description of the phenomenon.

◆ Literature review is an important component.

◆ In attempting to understand all aspects of a phenomenon, phenomenology equates with a philosophy of midwifery that emphasizes individual and holistic care.

REFERENCES

Annells M 1996 Hermeneutic phenomenology: philosophical perspectives and current use in nursing research. Journal of Advanced Nursing 23(4): 705–713

Baker C, Wuest J, Stern N 1992 Method slurring: the grounded theory/phenomenology example. Journal of Advanced Nursing 17(6): 1355–1360

Banonis B C 1989 The lived experience of recovering from addiction: a phenomenological study. Nursing Science Quarterly 2(1): 37–42

Beck C T 1994 Women's temporal experiences during the delivery process: a phenomenological study. International Journal of Nursing Studies 31(3): 245–252

Benner P 1994 Interpretative phenomenology – embodiment caring and ethics in health and illness. Sage Publications, Newbury Park, CA

Berg M, Dahlberg K 1998 A phenomenological study of women's experiences of complicated childbirth. Midwifery 14(1): 23–29

Bottorff J L 1990 Persistence in breastfeeding: a phenomenological investigation. Journal of Advanced Nursing 15(1): 201–209

Burns N, Grove S K 1993 The practice of nursing research, 2nd edn. WB Saunders, Philadelphia, PA

Clarke J B, Wheeler S J 1992 A view of the phenomenon of caring in nursing practice. Journal of Advanced Nursing 17(6): 1283–1290

Cohen M Z 1987 A historical overview of the phenomenologic movement. Image: Journal of Nursing Scholarship 19(1): 31–34

Colaizzi P 1978 Psychological research as the phenomenologist views it. In: Valle R, King M (ed) Existential phenomenological alternatives for psychology. Oxford University Press, Oxford

DePoy E, Gitlin L N 1994 Introduction to research. Mosby/Year Book, St Louis, MO

Donnison J 1988 Midwives and medical men. Historical Publications, London

Fielding N 1994 Varieties of research interviews. Nurse Researcher 1(3): 4–13

Garrett A 1982 Interviewing: its principles and methods. Family Service Association of America, New York

Gelis J 1991 History of childbirth. Polity Press, Cambridge

Giorgi A 1970 Psychology as a human science: a phenomenologically based approach. Harper & Row, New York

Giorgi A 1985 Phenomenology and psychological research. Duquesne University Press, Pittsburgh, PA

Guba E, Lincoln Y 1989 Fourth generation evaluation. Sage Publications, Newbury Park, CA

Halldorsdottir S, Karlsdottir S I 1996 Journeying through labour and delivery: perceptions of women who have given birth. Midwifery 12(1): 48–61

Holloway I, Wheeler S 1996 Qualitative research for nurses. Blackwell Science, Oxford

Holmes C A 1996 The politics of phenomenological concepts in nursing. Journal of Advanced Nursing 24(3): 579–587

Husserl E 1967 Ideas: general introduction to pure phenomenology. George Allen & Unwin, London

Jasper M A 1994 Issues in phenomenology for researchers of nursing. Journal of Advanced Nursing 19(2): 309–314

Koch T 1994 Establishing rigour in qualitative research: the decision trail. Journal of Advanced Nursing 19(5): 976–986

Lincoln Y S, Guba E G 1985 Naturalistic inquiry. Sage Publications, Newbury Park, CA

Lundgren I, Dahlberg K 1998 Women's experience of pain during childbirth. Midwifery 14(2): 105–110

Mills C 1994 Phenomenology. Surgical Nurse 7: 27–29

Morse J M 1992 Qualitative health research. Sage Publications, Newbury Park, CA

Morse J M, Field P A 1996 Nursing research: the application of qualitative approaches. Chapman & Hall, London

Oiler C 1982 The phenomenological approach in nursing research. Nursing Research 31(3): 178–181

Oleske D M, Heinze S, Otte D M 1990 The diary as a means of understanding the quality of life of persons with cancer receiving home nursing care. Cancer Nursing 13(3): 158–166

Omery A 1983 Phenomenology: a method for nursing research. Advances in Nursing Science January: 49–63

Paley J 1998 Misinterpretive phenomenology: Heidegger, ontology and nursing research. Journal of Advanced Nursing 27(4): 817–824

Patton M Q 1990 Qualitative evaluation and research methods, 2nd ed. Sage Publications, Newbury Park, CA

Polit D F, Hungler B P 1997 Nursing research – methods, appraisal, and utilization, 4th edn. JB Lippincott, Philadelphia, PA

Powers B A, Knapp T R 1995 A dictionary of nursing theory and research. Sage Publications, Thousand Oaks, CA

Reed J 1994 Phenomenology without phenomena: a discussion of the use of phenomenology to examine expertize in long-term care of elderly patients. Journal of Advanced Nursing 19(3): 336–341

Richardson A 1994 The health diary: an examination of its use as a data collection method. Journal of Advanced Nursing 19(4): 782–791

Robinson A 1995 The experiences of mothers breastfeeding term twins. Unpublished MSc thesis, University of Surrey

Robson C 1993 Real world research. Blackwell, Oxford

Rose K 1994 Unstructured and semi-structured interviewing. Nurse Researcher 1(3): 23–32

Roughman K, Haggerty R 1972 The diary as a research instrument in the study of health and illness behaviours. Medical Care 10(2): 143–163

Spiegelberg H 1965 The phenomenological movement: a historical introduction, vol 1, 2nd edn. Martinus Nijhoff, The Hague

Stewart D, Mickunas A 1990 Exploring phenomenology: a guide to the field and its literature. Ohio University Press, Athens, OH

Streubert H J, Carpenter D R 1999 Qualitative research in nursing: advancing the humanistic imperative, 2nd edn. Lippincott, Philadelphia

Talbot L A 1995 Principles and practice of nursing research. C V Mosby, St Louis, MO

Van Kaam A L 1959 Phenomenological analysis: exemplified by a study of the experience of 'really feeling understood'. Individual Psychology 15: 6–72

Walters A J 1995 The phenomenological movement: implications for nursing research. Journal of Advanced Nursing 22(4): 791–799

Winter R 1989 Learning from experience: principles and practices in action research. Falmer Press, Philadelphia, PA

9

Alternative approaches to research

Patricia Donovan

KEY ISSUES

◆ Integrating quantitative and qualitative approaches
◆ Triangulation
◆ Historical research
◆ Feminist approaches
◆ Action research
◆ Case studies

INTRODUCTION

Previous chapters of this book have explored the main research approaches but these may not meet the needs of an ever-evolving health-care system, the desire for new knowledge and a commitment to evidence-based practice. This chapter considers some of the newer and/or alternative approaches. They each use a multitude of data collecting methods in order to come to a conclusion, and how they do so depends on the philosophical and methodological stance of the researcher, who influences the research design. There is an increasing awareness of how both quantitative and qualitative methods can contribute to the study of midwifery. Ways of mixing quantitative and qualitative methods will be considered, focusing on triangulation, historical research, feminist approaches, action and evaluation research and case studies. Some of these, such as action research, are becoming more popular in nursing, but few midwives have adopted them. It is therefore difficult to provide midwifery examples and so, where possible, social and educational ones are given in their place. The discussion of each approach will attempt to take into account the perspective of the researcher, the clinical setting and in some cases the client. Both philosophical and practical considerations will be explored.

INTEGRATING QUANTITATIVE AND QUALITATIVE APPROACHES

There is controversy concerning the integration of qualitative and quantitative approaches. This is because of the underlying epistemological position from which each has developed. Hekman (1990) believes that there is a need for different methodologies because the goal of natural science, which is explanation, differs from the goal of social sciences, which is understanding. Midwifery, however, can be seen to be a combination of social sciences and natural sciences. Even within one study there may be one goal or aim, but this could be divided into individual objectives that incorporate explanation and understanding. This is analogous to holistic care. If midwives are to give individualized care there is a need to use different research approaches in order to further midwives' knowledge, understanding and future practice. Which approaches are chosen will depend on the goal of the research study.

Midwifery is an eclectic discipline and would benefit from an eclectic approach to developing and testing theory. Such an approach does not, however, seem to have developed. This may be because of the continuing debate between the polarized biomedical model of care and the woman-centred model, which has gained credibility nationally with the publication of the Winterton (Department of Health 1992) and *Changing Childbirth* (Department of Health 1993) reports.

Bryman (1992) lists 12 ways of integrating research approaches that have been identified in published reports. Steckler et al (1992) have incorporated these into four models, as shown in Box 9.1.

These models have led to a blurring of the boundaries between differing approaches. This offers advantages for midwifery research or any research into the maternity services that endeavours to provide an efficient and cost-effective service and one that meets the needs of clients. The most documented integration of approaches is seen in **triangulation** and this is now described in more detail.

TRIANGULATION

Triangulation has its origins in navigation and surveying. It then became a

Box 9.1 Integrating research approaches: four models (Steckler et al 1992, p. 5)

Model 1: Qualitative methods that are used to help develop quantitative measures and instruments

Model 2: Qualitative methods that are used to help explain quantitative findings

Model 3: Quantitative methods that are used to embellish a primarily qualitative study

Model 4: Qualitative and quantitative methods that are used equally and in parallel (this is the model that is usually regarded as triangulation)

Box 9.2 Types of triangulation (Denzin 1978)

◆ **Theoretical triangulation** uses different frames of reference or different perspectives to analyse the same data

◆ **Data triangulation** uses different sampling strategies to test theory in more than one way

◆ **Investigator triangulation** uses different people to observe, code, interview or analyse data in a study

◆ **Methodological triangulation** uses two or more methods of data collection within a study

quantitative technique, using two measurements to gain information about a variable. More recently it has come to mean the mixing of quantitative and qualitative approaches. There are four recognized types of triangulation, as shown in Box 9.2.

Triangulation can be seen as a means of overcoming the dichotomy between quantitative and qualitative approaches. It can be made as complex as desired and more than one type of triangulation can be undertaken in a study (Jones 1996). Gregory and McKie (1996) used discussion groups and questionnaires for their study on women's views of the cervical smear test. This type of triangulation appears most frequently in the literature. It is, however, important to remember that when methods are mixed they should always be appropriate to the research question. Triangulation can then increase the validity of a study.

There are three strategies associated with triangulation:

◆ within approach

◆ between approach
◆ combined.

The within approach or strategy is a combination of two or more data collection methods from the same approach, in the same study, in order to measure the same variable. An example of this could be the use of two quantitative scales in order to measure the same variables and then to compare the results. Denzin (1978) criticizes this, as it is still using quantitative measures rather than a mix of quantitative and qualitative approaches. The between approach is more popular because it combines quantitative and qualitative measures, as seen in the study by Gregory and McKie (1996). The combined strategy uses both of the previous strategies.

Triangulation is increasingly evident in nursing research but has yet to make any major contribution to midwifery. Nolan and Behi (1995) consider the concept of triangulation in more detail and you may find it helpful to refer to their text.

HISTORICAL RESEARCH

Midwifery research attempts to seek the truth but it could be argued that it will only uncover truth from one perspective. Midwifery is a practice-based profession and should be viewed within its context, which has evolved over generations influenced by the role of women in society.

Midwifery, like nursing, is considered to be of low status in comparison with professions such as medicine. However, midwifery predates medicine and other occupations and the old adage that 'midwifery is the second oldest profession' is still postulated. A historical perspective can therefore add to the current body of midwifery knowledge. Cultures value tradition passed down from one generation to the next, and one way of doing this is in the written form. **Historical research** may involve obtaining information from interviews as well as from archival material. The main historical texts are always written from the perspective of the 'winner' and obstetric histories are not exempt from this. Historical research takes into account the sociological, political and economic developments that shape the world at any particular time. It is therefore essential that midwives engage in historical research so that the hitherto unheard female voice can be not only heard but also given credence. When engaging in this type of research, there needs to be a defined focus, such as a person, as in the history of Dame Rosalind Paget written by John Rivers (1981), a place, as in the history of High Coombe (Beckett 1990), or a wider aspect such as the struggle for control of childbirth (Donnison 1988, Cowell 1981, Hannam 1996). Such works give inspiration and enable lessons to be learnt, especially for those countries that are experiencing a re-emergence of the midwifery profession. The dilemmas that were faced in this country by the emerging midwifery profession and its fight for legislation prior to the Midwives Act 1902 are not very different from dilemmas currently facing midwives in north America.

It is essential that researchers know how to analyse and interpret written texts, taking into account how and when they were produced. Some of the very first texts were written by midwives, even though the majority were illiterate. Different styles of writing may cause problems with interpreting the words used and what they mean within the context. Hallett (1997) refers to this in relation to nursing research and the difficulties she experienced in looking at nursing through medicine. The development of the midwifery profession was closely linked to the emergence of the obstetrician, who was originally a male midwife. Therefore, historical research into midwifery is difficult to extricate from the literature of the time. It is ironic that historically midwives have more in common with obstetricians than with nurses.

McGann (1997) discusses the first steps of historical research, which are defining the subject area and locating records. These records may include:

◆ public records
◆ hospital records
◆ local government records
◆ training and education
◆ nursing/midwifery associations
◆ private papers
◆ journals
◆ books.

How the midwife was portrayed in the media of the time may also be useful to historians and no historical midwifery text seems to be free of Dickens's Sarah Gamp (Hughes 1990).

Once the data is collected it must be interpreted and this can be a mammoth task. When analysing texts written by others it is worth remembering that the researcher is interpreting another person's interpretation. This is known as the **double hermeneutic** and needs to be taken into account. Vital elements in this process are the objectivity, judgement and creativity of the researcher (Kerr 1986). Most historical research, like ethnographies, is published in the form of books and it is possibly because of this that readers are not always aware that they are reading research!

FEMINIST APPROACHES

Feminist research is any research that is conducted by feminists or by those who knowingly or unknowingly adopt a feminist perspective or feminist criteria. As midwifery can be viewed from a feminist perspective, it is appropriate to consider the role of feminist research in midwifery. Midwifery can be viewed from a feminist perspective either as an extension of the work of mothers and midwives or as a skilled practitioner. Etzioni (1969) believed that women in a female occupation would engage in trivial discourse about personal matters and be unable to be objective or exercise authority. This reinforces the concept that objectivity, scientific approaches and the medical viewpoint are masculine and hence the predominant research domain is masculine. This implies that feminism has no place in research, but this is excluding a potentially important perspective on all research, particularly where the majority of participants are women, as in midwifery.

Male-defined models of knowledge and ways of accessing knowledge are identified by Gunew (1990). This implies there must also be female-defined models of knowledge and female ways of accessing it. Viewed from a feminist perspective it could be argued that, within a female occupation, knowledge and its acquisition should adopt a feminine model. This would take a subjective view of women and is consistent with the concept of midwife being 'with woman'. Feminist research is about articulating these differences and helping midwives to adopt the feminine model, as previously they have been criticized for being agents of the medical model, transforming childbirth into a medical ritual (Barclay et al 1989).

All research embodies and enacts power relations. This is because research involves the researcher and the researched. Data collection and analysis are not neutral acts, they are acts involving power. This is closely related to gender questions and the whole question of feminist research. Fonow and Cook (1991) suggest that the male voice defines the self in terms of distinctness and separation from others. The female voice defines the self in terms of connections and relationships. This view is applied to the quantitative/qualitative debate, with the conclusion that the female voice is qualitative. Oakley (1993, p. 245), in talking about feminist research and the research process, states that 'it should not employ methods oppressive either to researchers or to the researched, and... it should be oriented towards the production of knowledge in such a form and in such a way as can be used for women themselves'. These, she states, are also criteria for good research.

Researchers may choose methods of data collection that they can control, such as structured questionnaires. Control is a gendered concept. Qualitative methods, such as interviewing, can also be viewed as masculine. Oakley (1981) considers interviewing women a contradiction in terms. She believes that interviewing controls women as the interviewer asks the questions and not the women. Therefore, qualitative methods of data collection are not necessarily feminine and helpful to women. Oakley decided that as a feminist she would answer any questions concerning the research or herself. However, this does not mean the exclusion of all quantitative approaches from feminist research. Oakley (1993) identified that some researchers have argued that quantitative research results in the domination of the research process over the participants. She, however, was able to combine a feminist philosophy with a randomized control trial in her study of social support (Oakley 1992). Oakley (1993) therefore succeeds in destroying the myth that qualitative methods of data collection are exclusively 'feminine' and vice versa. Methods themselves do not appear to have gender – it is the way they are used and the purpose that they are used for.

To ensure that research itself is not gendered, researchers need to be reflexive as to the motive of their research as well as the motivation behind the selection of specific methods of data collection. They also have to question how they relate to the researched and to make explicit the power relations that exist within the study. The acknowledgment of a degree of control can have the ability to reduce the controlling element to some extent. It should be noted that research methods are sometimes dictated by those who are funding the research. Oakley (1993) had a difficult time gaining funding for her research on social support in pregnancy. This was because those who provided funding lacked an understanding of feminist research.

There are many feminist perspectives, ranging from liberal through conservative, social to radical. Webb (1993) attempts to list the characteristics of feminist research (Box 9.3).

Box 9.3 The characteristics of feminist research according to Webb (1993)

◆ The researcher is a woman.
◆ Feminist methodology is used, which includes interaction with subjects, expression of feelings and concern for values.
◆ The research has the potential to help its subjects (women).
◆ The focus is on the experiences of women.
◆ The words feminism or feminist are used.
◆ Feminist literature is cited.
◆ The research is reported using nonsexist language.

However, it is important to remember that a feminist who adopts a feminist approach regardless of the needs of the topic area being studied could be considered biased from the outset. Midwives are in a prime position to perform feminist research (Draper 1997) and yet few have done so. This may be because research is new to midwives and the majority of role models have been from the male scientific community, which has resulted in midwives adopting a male rather than a feminist perspective. This may be associated with midwifery's efforts to gain recognition and equal status alongside obstetricians. Alternatively, midwives may have undertaken feminist research but not recognized it or labelled it as feminist.

ACTION RESEARCH

Action research was first proposed as a method of enquiry nearly 50 years ago by Kurt Lewin. One aspect of Lewin's thinking was the symbiotic relationship between theory and practice, and action research was designed to bridge the perceived gap between theory and practice (Lewin 1946).

Action research has become increasingly popular within practice-based professions such as education and nursing. This may be because of continuing efforts to reduce the theory–practice gap. This perceived gap has been researched in midwifery in recent times (Donovan 1994, 1996) but few midwifery studies have adopted an action research approach.

Elliott (1991, p. 49) states that 'the fundamental aim of action research is to improve practice rather than to produce knowledge'. It is therefore an ideal method for midwives to use as they should always be striving to improve their practice. The implementation of the *Changing Childbirth* report (Department of Health 1993) recommendations could have been explored using an action research approach; however other approaches were deemed to be more effective.

Greenwood (1994) defines three main approaches to action research, depending on the underlying philosophical basis, but they all include the following characteristics, described by Holter and Schwartz-Barcott (1993):

◆ collaboration between researcher and practitioner
◆ solution of practical problems
◆ change in practice
◆ development of theory.

The action research cycle is similar to the nursing process or any problem solving approach and is outlined below:

Assessment – Planning – Action – Evaluation

This indicates a straightforward linear approach. However, the reality of action research is that assessment and planning may be revisited prior to the action stage. Cohen and Manion (1989) discuss eight stages (Box 9.4), and these would appear to reflect the reality of the process.

Obtaining ethical approval may be difficult in this type of study because of the collaborative nature of the process. Ethics Committees tend to have a

Box 9.4 Stages of the action research cycle (Cohen and Manion 1989)

Stage 1 – Identification of the problem. In this stage the problem that is seen in the everyday situation is identified, evaluated and further defined. The term 'problem' may be seen as detrimental to midwifery, which views childbirth as a normal process. 'Need' is therefore substituted for 'problem'. Whichever terminology is used, the issue or focus of the research is identified.

Stage 2 – Discussion. Discussion takes place among interested and involved parties and from this a research proposal may be formulated.

Stage 3 – Literature review. A literature review is undertaken, which reviews other studies, and an exploration of the need or issue may take place in the light of other research findings.

Stage 4 – Redefinition of the need. At this stage the need may be revisited in a similar way to stage 1, taking into account all the findings of previous stages. A hypothesis may be developed or a set of guiding principles. Any assumptions underlying the project are made explicit.

Stage 5 – Research procedures. Selection of research procedures, sampling and deployment of the people involved is decided.

Stage 6 – Choice of evaluation procedures. How the action or change is evaluated is decided.

Stage 7 – Implementation and stage 8 – Interpretation of data. These last two stages are self-explanatory.

greater understanding of quantitative methods with set procedures and protocols. Action research may change and evolve as the study continues and those in practice develop the process and refine it. The process is therefore difficult to predict and this may produce problems for those on Ethics Committees. A dynamic, practice-led research study may reach aims and conclusions that may not have been thought of at the commencement of the work.

EVALUATION RESEARCH

Evaluation research has only become known as a form of research in the last 25 years. In the National Health Service evaluation is important because of the increasing focus on managerial and resource accountability. The purposes of evaluation research include:

◆ accrediting educational programmes
◆ informing decision-making

- ✦ seeing what works
- ✦ legitimating sponsored educational programmes
- ✦ gaining a holistic understanding.

As a result of the *Changing Childbirth* report (Department of Health 1993), there have been a number of pilot studies set up to provide continuity of care. Following the initiation of these studies evaluation has taken place in a number of localities (Turnbull et al 1995). One of the main reasons for attempting evaluation of these studies was to establish whether the pilot schemes should continue, and in doing so become accepted examples of good practice. In this way evaluation informs decision making and 'stake-holders' who ultimately control their funding. In a health service where directorates are constantly competing for limited resources evaluation is a means of justifying the care that is given.

Three main categories of evaluation research are identified by MacDonald (1987; Box 9.5).

Box 9.5 Categories of action research (MacDonald 1987)

- ✦ **Bureaucratic evaluations** play an instrumental role in maintaining and extending managerial power. The evaluator holds the same values as those in managerial power. The 'reality of power' is the implicit rationale of bureaucratic evaluations — evaluation for hire.

- ✦ **Autocratic evaluations** maintain and extend power by offering scientific legitimacy to public policy in exchange for compliance with the evaluator's recommendations. The power base is with the academic community, who retain ownership of the strategy. The final report may be held by the bureaucracy but is also published in academic journals. Objectivity and distancing from the power base is maintained.

- ✦ **Democratic evaluations** give power to those at the forefront of the evaluation, the participants or informants. These informants control the evaluation information. Periodic negotiation of the evaluator's relationship with the sponsors and programme participants takes place throughout the study. Key concepts appear to be confidentiality, negotiation and accessibility.

The commonest form of evaluation is autocratic. Sponsors and 'stake-holders' may be the English National Board, who commission evaluations, or individual NHS Trusts, who support evaluation of specific programmes that have been instigated by them or the Department of Health.

You might question whether evaluation is research. Evaluation is usually part of any programme of learning as it is part of the midwifery or nursing care process cycle. All practitioners need to evaluate their practice, whether it involves specific advice to a client or a teaching session or educational course. When systematic evaluation is done, preferably by outsiders in order to uncover and explore the project or role, it can be considered as research. There are many studies that could be described as evaluation research but do not use that terminology. Studies that have explored specific roles such as Advanced Neonatal Nurse Practitioner (Redshaw and Harris 1995, Dillon and George 1997) as well as midwives (Robinson et al 1983), and studies that have looked at courses and means of preparing midwives (Mander 1989, Fraser 1996) could all be considered evaluative in nature. Evaluation studies classified as bureaucratic, autocratic or democratic uncover the power bases, which may otherwise not be explicit.

Murphy-Black (1991), discussing evaluation of a postbasic training course, used a tripartite **Donabedian approach** that focused on structure, process and outcome. Midwifery journals provide examples of evaluation projects that have arisen following the *Changing Childbirth* report (Department of Health 1993). 'Team midwifery', 'midwifery-led care' and 'midwifery development units' have all been evaluated (Turnbull et al 1995). Ness (1998) suggests that purchasers and providers need reliable information concerning existing services before initiating change. Only then can the impact of change be evaluated.

Evaluation studies can be confused with action research. Action research is mainly collaborative and more dynamic than evaluation research, which will have 'stake-holders' external to the process. Ness (1998) took part in a project to evaluate change in three maternity units, the findings of which are as yet unpublished. This report highlighted the financial constraints and questioned some of the recommendations of *Changing Childbirth* (Department of Health 1993). This could be viewed as bureaucratic evaluation because the report, which has been submitted to the Department of Health, has not yet been published as it questions present policy. There is a place for democratic evaluation within midwifery but not when 'stake-holders' control the findings. If a service is to be women-centred, evaluation of such a service must also be in the control of women, irrespective of who the funding agent is.

CASE STUDIES

The case study viewed from a quantitative perspective has briefly been referred to in Chapter 3. Case studies can also be explored using a qualitative approach. Alternatively, as what is being studied can often be viewed from different perspectives: triangulation can be adopted. According to Holloway and Wheeler (1996), case studies have a clearly determined focus such as an individual, a group or a particular setting and it is this that distinguishes them from other qualitative approaches. The emphasis is on studying one unit. This could be one midwife, a specific group of midwives, such as independent midwives, or a general practitioner unit or teaching hospital. There are no differences in the way data is collected and analysed and, as Stake (1998, p. 86) notes, 'the case study is not a methodological choice, but a choice of object to be studied. We choose to study the case.' Stake (1998) refers to three types of case study although he acknowledges that there are others (Box 9.6).

Box 9.6 Types of case study (Stake 1998)

- ◆ **Intrinsic case study:** one in which the researcher has a particular interest and wishes to enhance her/his knowledge and understanding. These are evident in medical journals where a particular illness or structural malformation which is rarely seen is studied. This parallels the quantitative approach to case studies.
- ◆ **Instrumental case study,** where the case study helps the researcher to understand another issue.
- ◆ **Collective case study,** which is an instrumental case study that explores a number of cases.

It is important to remember that findings are of a typical or atypical case. A typical case may have characteristics some of which are recognized as common to other cases. However, viewed within a specific context, these characteristics cannot be transferred or generalized to a whole population. The atypical case, according to Stake (1998), limits the extent to which the findings of other cases can be generalized by drawing attention to alternative characteristics. Midwives, for example, are usually viewed as being caring health practitioners. An atypical or negative example would be the midwife who bullies or intimidates the women s/he cares for and other midwives with whom s/he works. By establishing the variations or dimensions within a theme, theory can be refined or extended.

CONCLUSION

This chapter has provided an overview of research approaches that are not commonly seen in medical, nursing or midwifery research. Action research is a developing approach because of its collaborative and flexible nature. Many of these research approaches endeavour to expose the underlying power base, which is present in all forms of research but seldom discussed. As midwifery knowledge develops through the process of research, researchers will feel able to explore and develop knowledge using the approaches discussed in this chapter and not limit themselves to those imposed by other professional groups.

CHAPTER SUMMARY

This chapter has highlighted:

The main approaches to research do not always need the needs of the researcher or the topic to be explored. Alternative approaches include:

◆ Historical research

◆ Action research

◆ Evaluation research

◆ Feminist approaches

◆ Case studies.

To ensure goals are achieved it will sometimes be appropriate to integrate quantitative and qualitative approaches.

REFERENCES

Barclay L, Andre C, Glover P 1989 Women's business: the challenge of childbirth. Midwifery 5(3): 122–133

Beckett E 1990 History of High Coombe 1950–1986. Council of the Midwife Teachers Training College, Surbiton

Bryman A 1992 Quantitative and qualitative research: further reflections on their integration. In: Brannen J (ed) Mixing methods: qualitative and quantitative research. Avebury, Aldershot, p 57–78

Cohen L, Manion L 1989 Research methods in education, 3rd edn. Croom Helm, Beckenham

Cowell B 1981 Behind the blue door: the history of the Royal College of Midwives. Baillière Tindall, London

Denzin N K 1978 The research act: a theoretical introduction to sociological methods. McGraw-Hill, New York

Department of Health 1992 Maternity services. Health Committee Second Report. HMSO, London

Department of Health 1993 Changing childbirth. The report of the Expert Committee, vol 1. HMSO, London

Dillon A, George S 1997 Advanced neonatal practitioners in the United Kingdom: where are they and what do they do? Journal of Advanced Nursing 25(2): 257–264

Donnison J 1988 Midwives and medical men, 2nd edn. Historical Publications Ltd., London

Donovan P 1994 A study of practice based education. University of Southampton, Unpublished MAEd Thesis

Donovan P 1996 The practice theory gap in midwifery. Southampton University, MPhil Unpublished Thesis

Draper J 1997 Potential and problems: the value of feminist approaches to research. British Journal of Medicine 5(10): 597–600

Elliott J 1991 Action research for educational change. Open University, Milton Keynes

Etzioni A 1969 The semi-professions and their organisations. Free Press, New York

Fonow M M, Cook J A 1991 Beyond methodology: feminist scholarship as lived research. Indiana University Press, Bloomington, IN

Fraser D 1996 Preregistration midwifery programmes: a case study evaluation of the non-midwifery placements. Midwifery 12(1): 16–22

Greenwood J 1994 Action research and action researchers: some introductory considerations. Contemporary Nurse 3: 84–92

Gregory S, McKie L 1996 Negotiation and compromise in researching women's views of the cervical smear test. In: McKie L (ed) Researching women's health. Mark Allen Publications, Salisbury

Gunew S (ed) 1990 Feminist knowledge. Routledge, London

Hallett C 1997 Historical texts: factors affecting their interpretation. Nurse Researcher 5(2): 61–70

Hannam J 1996 Some aspects of the history of the Royal College of Midwives. In: Robinson S, Thomson A (ed) Midwives, research and childbirth, vol 4. Chapman & Hall, London, ch 2, p 10–33

Hekman S J 1990 Gender and knowledge: elements of a postmodern feminism. Polity Press, Cambridge

Holloway I, Wheeler S 1996 Qualitative research for nurses. Blackwell Science, Oxford

Holter I M, Schwartz-Barcott D 1993 Action research: what is it? How has it been used and how can it be used in nursing? Journal of Advanced Nursing 18(2): 298–304

Hughes D 1990 Sarah Gamp – midwife. ARM Midwifery Matters 66: 12

Jones W 1996 Triangulation in clinical practice. Journal of Clinical Nursing 5: 319–323

Kerr J 1986 Historical nursing research. In: Stinson S M, Kerr J (ed) International issues in nursing research, vol 1. Croom Helm, London, p 322

Lewin K 1946 Action Research and minority problems. Journal of Social Issues 2(4): 34–36

MacDonald B 1987 Evaluation and the control of education. In: Murphy R, Torrance H (ed) Evaluating education: issues and methods, vol 1. Open University, Milton Keynes, p 362

Mander R 1989 'The best laid schemes . . .': an evaluation of the extension of midwifery training in Scotland. International Journal Nursing Studies 27(1): 27–41

McGann S 1997 Archival sources for research into the history of nursing. Nurse Researcher 5(2): 19–29

Murphy-Black T 1991 Antenatal education: evaluation of a post-basic training course. In: Robinson S, Thomson A (ed) Midwives, research and childbirth, vol 2. Chapman & Hall, London, ch 7, p 176–199

Ness M 1998 Evaluation of midwifery services – a personal reflection. British Journal of Midwifery 6(1): 53–55

Nolan M, Behi R 1995 Triangulation: the best of all worlds? British Journal of Nursing 4(14): 829–832

Oakley A 1981 Interviewing women: a contradiction in terms. In: Roberts H (ed) Doing feminist research. RKP, London

Oakley A 1992 Social support in motherhood: the natural history of a research project. Blackwell, Oxford

Oakley A 1993 Women, medicine and health. Edinburgh University Press, Edinburgh

Redshaw M, Harris A 1995 Breaking new ground: an exploratory study of the role and education of the advanced neonatal nurse practitioner. Research Reports 4. English National Board, London

Rivers J 1981 Dame Rosalind Paget – a short account of her life and work. Midwives Chronicle, London

Robinson S, Golden J, Bradley S 1983 A study of the role and responsibilities of the midwife. Nursing Education Research Unit, Report No 1. Chelsea College, University of London, London

Stake R E 1998 Case studies. In: Denzin N K, Lincoln Y S (ed) Strategies of qualitative inquiry. Sage Publications, Thousand Oaks, CA, ch 4, p 86–109

Steckler A, McLeroy K, Goodman R, Bird S, McCormick L 1992 Towards integrating qualitative and quantitative methods: an introduction. Health Education Quarterly 19(1): 1–8

Turnbull D, McGinley M, Fyvie H et al 1995 Implementation and evaluation of a midwifery development unit. British Journal of Midwifery 3(9): 465–468

Webb C 1993 Feminist research: definitions, methodology, methods and evaluation. Journal of Advanced Nursing 18(3): 416–423

10

Critiquing the literature

Rosalind Bluff   Elizabeth Cluett

KEY ISSUES

◆ The elements of a critique including:
  – title, authors and the journal
  – the abstract
  – the literature review
  – the approach and method
  – the findings
  – the discussion and implications
◆ Validity, reliability and trustworthiness
◆ Ethical issues
◆ Conclusions from a critique

INTRODUCTION

The need to base midwifery practice on available evidence has already been emphasized in this book. No research study is perfect because, for example, constraints are imposed on the researcher(s) by the clinical setting and ethical issues. Publication in a well-respected journal does not therefore necessarily mean it is a good piece of research. In previous chapters we have considered various research approaches. In this chapter we have integrated the knowledge you have gained of the quantitative and qualitative research processes and suggested some questions you might want to ask to effectively interpret a research study or report. The aim is to highlight the process of critiquing;

if necessary, you can refer back to previous chapters in the book for explanations and detail on aspects of the research process.

We have chosen to use the term **critique** rather than evaluation. Although both terms have been used synonymously (Rees 1994, Parahoo 1997), Leininger (1994) makes a distinction, and the lack of set criteria, which she argues are necessary for evaluation, suggests that critique is a more appropriate term to use. Similarity of the word critique to those of critic and criticism may lead to an assumption that only negative aspects of a study are identified. Critiquing, however, involves reviewing the literature in order to identify both strengths and weaknesses. In this way a judgement can be made about the value of the research study. On the basis of this judgement, one of a number of decisions can be made:

◆ to use the evidence to inform decision-making in clinical practice
◆ to reject the evidence on the basis of serious flaws in the research design
◆ to reserve judgement about the value of the research study until further research evidence confirms or refutes the findings.

Critical reading is a skill that can be developed (Price and Price 1996), but it does need to be practised regularly. Critiquing involves asking questions of all aspects of the research process. When formulating your questions you may find it helpful to consider the use of prefixes such as where, when, what, why and how. You may find it useful to obtain a research study so that, as you work through this chapter, you can apply the knowledge gained from it. Initially, you may need to read the article several times, focusing on different aspects of the study on each occasion.

Issues that need to be addressed when critiquing the literature are explored under appropriate headings. However, you will find that some research studies amalgamate several issues under one heading.

TITLE

The title of a research study should reflect the content of the study and be clear and concise. 'A study on the effects of low haemoglobin on postnatal women' (Paterson et al 1994) provides a clear indication of what the research study is about. In contrast, the title 'Midwives' burnout and continuity of care' (Sandall 1997), although concise, does lack clarity. The content of this article identifies continuity of carer as the cause of midwives' burnout. Although the provision of continuity of carer aims to provide continuity of care these are nevertheless separate issues. This highlights the importance of careful and precise use of words to convey the meaning intended.

AUTHORS

Individuals who undertake research should have the necessary skills to fulfil the aims and objectives of the study. Readers need to ascertain who the researchers are, whether they have relevant qualifications and if they were appropriate individuals to undertake the research study. If the research study is related to maternity care but the researchers are not midwives this does not mean they are inappropriate people to carry out the research. If you are not sure of their appropriateness your decision may be based on your judgement of the value of the study when the critique is completed. A poorly designed study with major flaws might suggest an inexperienced researcher with inadequate supervision, researchers who lack the skills for the particular methods they have adopted or a nonmidwife researcher who lacks the appropriate professional knowledge.

You may be familiar with the names of some researchers but others you will not know. Researchers sometimes collaborate with each other and it can be helpful to ascertain if they are linked to a research unit. For example, you may not know the researchers but some or all of them may work for the National Perinatal Epidemiology Unit, a well-respected unit that specializes in research associated with maternity care. It is also useful to look at the skills each researcher brings to a study. A statistician, epidemiologist and economist all have skills that potentially enhance the quality of the study.

JOURNAL

A number of journals publish research studies. Midwives need to consider whether the journal is an appropriate one for publishing the article they are critiquing. The journal *Midwifery*, for example, focuses on studies carried out by midwives or by those undertaking studies related to maternity care. A pilot study of pushing in the second stage of labour (Thomson 1993) was published in the *Journal of Advanced Nursing*. One might question whether this journal was appropriate when few clinical midwives were likely to access it with the expectation of finding an article of relevance to their clinical practice.

Most journals now have articles reviewed by one or two experienced researchers from the same discipline as the researchers who have undertaken the study. Nevertheless, this is something you need to look for. The information is sometimes to be found in the instructions to contributors. When the research study has been peer reviewed this suggests that a certain standard of work must be achieved before publication will be considered. Experimental research studies will only be published in the *British Journal of Obstetrics and Gynaecology* if they meet specified criteria (Grant 1995).

ABSTRACT

An abstract should provide a comprehensive summary of the research study and in doing so rectify any deficiencies in the title. The purpose of the study should be stated, together with the methods adopted and the main findings (Parahoo 1997). When referring to databases the clarity of the abstract may be particularly important if the study is not readily available and a charge is made by the library to obtain the article. Ideally, it should be presented in an interesting format to encourage further reading and it must be accurate, as some practitioners may rely on the abstract for information rather than reading the complete article.

LITERATURE REVIEW/JUSTIFICATION FOR STUDY

A comprehensive literature review provides the means by which the researcher(s) can justify the area of investigation and the selected research design, particularly if the design has been based on earlier studies and/or modifications have been undertaken to meet the needs of this specific study. It is important to remember that a research article cannot be viewed in isolation. It needs to be placed in context with other literature on the topic. A summary of what is known on the topic should be provided and this knowledge should be related to the area of the researcher's investigation. When a research report is presented in full, as in a dissertation or book, you can expect the literature review to be more extensive than that found in a journal article. In either case, there should be evidence of a logical structure, both of the main topic and of any issues that arise directly from it. The researcher should critique the literature and in this way the importance of the study can be identified. Gaps in knowledge or flaws in previous research designs should be revealed, and the contribution this study will make to the existing body of knowledge highlighted. As well as literature related specifically to midwifery you also need to consider whether the researchers have explored the application of relevant concepts, theories or frameworks from other relevant disciplines such as nursing, medicine, physiotherapy, sociology or haematology to their own work.

You will need to undertake your own literature search to ascertain if all relevant literature on the topic has been considered. This does not have to be as extensive as if you were undertaking the study yourself. You might begin by considering the researcher's reference list or using one or more of the literature sources identified in Chapter 3. By gaining access to some of this material you can critique it yourself. Note the ratio between primary and secondary sources of literature. Ideally, primary sources should predominate unless there is difficulty gaining access to them. Reference should be made to current research and texts, but it can be appropriate to refer to older material. For example, in studies which adopt a grounded theory approach you would expect 'The discovery of grounded theory' (Glaser and Strauss 1967) to be referenced, as this is a seminal text. Pocock 1983 is a classic text for those undertaking clinical trials.

It is incumbent on the reader to consider the research issue from alternative perspectives. Bias may be evident if literature presented supports only one view of the research topic. It is possible that only this view is represented in the literature, but the researcher should acknowledge this.

THE RESEARCH TOPIC

The purpose of the research study should be clearly stated. In experimental research you will need to look for a hypothesis or null hypothesis. Sometimes subhypotheses are also stated. Nonexperimental quantitative research studies are associated with a research question or objectives. These should all provide a clear focus for the study. De Jong et al (1997, p. 567), in a randomized control trial, do not overtly state a hypothesis but an objective is stated in the abstract to the study: 'to assess the maternal and neonatal effects of upright compared with recumbent positions during delivery, in terms of defined outcome variables'. This study is clearly about maternal position during labour. It can be assumed this refers to the second stage of labour, although this is stated in the title of the study and not the objective. The objective does not make clear what type of effects the researchers were looking for or the outcome measures, for example pain levels, maternal satisfaction or physiological parameters such as blood loss, cardiotocographic responses of the fetus or neonatal blood gases. These issues are revealed in the main body of the article but if a precise statement of the objectives had clearly set out the research goals it might have been easier to identify whether they had been achieved.

Having ensured that the research questions or hypotheses are clear you will need to check that you have identified and understood the research variables and possible outcomes. Remember, there may be dependent, independent and extraneous variables as well as primary and secondary out-comes to consider in quantitative studies. It is necessary for you to consider whether these have been explored in sufficient detail, particularly whether there are any extraneous variables that have not been controlled for.

You will also need to check your understanding of any terminology that is used. This should be unambiguous, particularly when it refers to variables. You should not have to make assumptions. 'Waterbirth', for example, could be interpreted to mean women giving birth in water or, alternatively, using the waterbirth pool only for relief of pain during the first stage of labour.

You would not expect qualitative studies to define the research question in the form of a hypothesis or objectives. These are contrary to the qualitative research process. The purpose of the study is usually expressed in the form of an aim because the study is initially broader than a quantitative one. Researchers avoid specifying the agenda in the form of objectives, because they may identify what is important to them rather than what is important to their participants. This could inhibit the process of discovery associated with qualitative research.

APPROACH

When critiquing a research study it is important to identify the approach adopted. This may be quantitative or qualitative. The reader needs to identify whether the selected approach was appropriate for the topic or phenomenon which was studied. For example, it would be appropriate to adopt a quantitative approach if one form of treatment or care option was being compared with another, such as upright versus supine position in labour (de Jong et al 1997). Qualitative research is appropriate for exploring thoughts, feelings and experiences and is particularly helpful when little is known about a topic (Glaser and Strauss 1967). Remember that the dynamic nature of qualitative research means that researchers adapt their approach to meet the needs of their study. They should, however, like quantitative researchers, provide sufficient information to demonstrate the process and justify what they have done. The depth of this may vary according to which journal the article is published in. *Midwifery* journal may make assumptions that readers already have some understanding of the research process and therefore provide less detail than other journals. Publishers also provide word limitations. Researchers therefore have to make decisions about which areas of their study to include in detail, what to exclude and what can be discussed at a superficial level. This means that their work is vulnerable to criticism by those who read it. Midwives undertaking research at Masters or PhD level are advised to obtain the primary source of the research study.

Some studies combine quantitative and qualitative methods. This may provide a comprehensive view of the research topic. There is, however, a lack of agreement about whether it is appropriate to do this (Holloway and Wheeler 1996). You may find it helpful to ask yourself what information was gained by using two approaches that could not have been obtained using one.

METHOD

We noted the difference between methodology and method in Chapter 2. Research protocol (Pocock 1983) or design (Polit and Hungler 1997, Arber 1993, Parahoo 1997) are sometimes used in place of the term 'method'. A rationale for the method should be included in the study. If a quantitative approach was adopted there should be enough information about the method to enable a similarly experienced researcher to replicate the study accurately. In a qualitative research study it must be remembered that the researcher is the research tool. The study cannot be replicated but the provision of an audit trail (Lincoln and Guba 1985) will help you to recognize how the theory was developed.

The most common quantitative methods are surveys, comparative studies and experimental studies. The key characteristics of an experiment are randomization, a control group and an intervention. The presence of a valid experimental research process must be carefully considered as part of the critique. Studies may be retrospective or prospective. Qualitative research studies include ethnography, phenomenology and grounded theory. All these approaches have been discussed in previous chapters of this book.

Method includes issues of sampling, data collection and analysis, validity, reliability or trustworthiness of the data and ethical issues, all of which will now be considered under their separate headings.

Sample

Sampling is a key issue, which, if inappropriate, will adversely influence the validity and reliability of a study. When considering the issue of sampling, size, characteristics, type of population, participation rate and selection will need to be addressed. The approach to sampling differs according to the approaches adopted and quantitative techniques are not considered appropriate for qualitative studies (Morse 1991). How individuals in the study are referred to may indicate the research background of the authors. Subjects are usually associated with quantitative research while participants or respondents are the preferred terms in qualitative studies. Inappropriate use of these terms may prompt the reader to question whether the author(s) has previously undertaken the approach adopted and is unfamiliar with the terminology or the research process.

Sample size

Samples selected by quantitative researchers tend to be large. This is because the aim is to accept or reject the hypothesis and/or generalize findings to the population as a whole. If you are critiquing a quantitative study you will need to check that the sample size is adequate for the chosen tests of significance. This may have been established using power calculations. A small sample size may indicate a pilot study. Further information on sample size can be found in Chapter 3. Sample sizes tend to be small in qualitative studies, although there are exceptions. This is because the strategies for data collection and analysis are very time-consuming and the amount of data collected can be considerable. The aim of qualitative research is, however, to gain insight into and understanding of a phenomenon or phenomena and not to generalize the findings. In a grounded theory study the sample size should be sufficient to achieve saturation of theoretical categories.

Sample criteria

It is important to identify characteristics of the sample. These should be the same in experimental and control groups. The aim is to avoid introducing bias into the study. The exact nature of the research study will determine which characteristics are vital, which are of interest and which are irrelevant. As the midwife critiquing the study you must use your clinical knowledge to judge whether all appropriate characteristics have been considered and how, if at all, these compare with your own practice environment. When considering the characteristics of the sample, you may find the subheadings in Box 10.1 useful, although in practice many of these issues are interdependent.

Box 10.1 Characteristics of the sample to be considered when critiquing

◆ **Global perspective,** e.g. ethnic origins, country research conducted in and health-care provision
◆ **National perspective,** e.g. regional variations in socio-economic status and educational levels.
◆ **Local environment,** e.g. rural or urban and employment opportunities.
In addition to these broad characteristics, specific defining features are usually identified within inclusion and/or exclusion criteria, such as parity or obstetric risk.

Morse (1991) acknowledges the need for the sample in any qualitative study to be appropriate and adequate for the aims of the study to be achieved. Characteristics of the sample are of interest because, for example, where a woman gives birth and her perception of the experience may be influenced by her socioeconomic group and the factors that influence this. However, it would be inappropriate to select the sample on the basis of their characteristics. To gain insight into a phenomenon, what is important is the participants' knowledge of the topic, hence the need for purposive sampling. Events, situations and concepts may also be sampled, not just individuals. Those excluded from qualitative studies should be identified and the reason for this should be given. The sample may appear biased because, for example, only women having a vaginal delivery and not those experiencing a caesarean section have been included in the study (Bluff and Holloway 1994).

The number of the selected sample who actually take part in the study, i.e. the participation rate, or the response rate in the case of questionnaires, also needs to be considered. There can be many reasons why the identified sample may not be accessed. Individuals may decline to participate. Whether it is a quantitative or qualitative study it is helpful to know the reasons for this. Notes may be lost but if the number of individuals is smaller than planned there is potential for bias to occur. This issue is included under the sample section for completeness, but is often reported as part of the research findings. It is always worth comparing intended sample details with the actual sample achieved.

Sample selection

How the sample is selected is important. Remember, the 'individual' may be an organization, a set of notes or an event, not just a person. The main methods of sampling selection for quantitative and qualitative research are summarized in Table 10.1. The authors should clearly state which method was chosen and why. Occasionally more than one method of sampling is used within one study.

Table 10.1 A summary of the methods of sample selection in quantitative and qualitative approaches

Quantitative approaches	Qualitative approaches
Probability sampling All individuals have a known chance of selection: • Simple • Stratified • Systematic • Cluster	**Purposive sampling** • Convenience • Open • Snowballing/chaining • Theoretical (grounded theory)
Nonprobability sampling The chance of any individual being selected is not known • Convenience/accidental	

The research environment

The context in which the research took place should be described. In qualitative research this influences participants' perceptions of the phenomenon being studied. In quantitative studies the physical environment may affect the biophysical parameters that are being measured. For example, it would be difficult for a researcher to measure the fundal height of a gravid uterus if it was too dark to see the tape measure. Qualitative researchers find field notes a valuable means of recording contextual data. If a good description of the research setting is provided, you may be left to make an assumption that such notes were kept.

Data collection

Readers need to know the strategies that were used for collecting data to determine whether they were appropriate. Look for biophysical measurements and event parameters such as length of labour, and structured questionnaires and interviews in quantitative studies. These should be supported with evidence on the accuracy and consistency of the measurements obtained (validity and reliability). There may also be detail of whether the data collection method has previously been used and is well known, such as the Edinburgh postnatal depression scale (Cox et al 1987). In qualitative research you would expect to find evidence of unstructured and semistructured interviews or participant and nonparticipant observation, or a combination of these. Davies (1996), for example, in a study that explored students' experiences of the first 18 weeks of their midwifery course, collected data using participant observation, individual interviews, group discussion, diaries completed by students and documents such as handouts given to students. The collection of data using a number of approaches is known as triangulation (Denzin 1978). The understanding of a phenomenon can be increased by the depth and detail obtained using several approaches. The trustworthiness of the data is also likely to be enhanced but the researcher should make clear to readers why these strategies were adopted. For example, they may overcome the possibility that what some individuals say they do in practice is not what they do in reality.

When critiquing how data was collected readers need to know when data was collected. Some studies take place over a prolonged period of time. The time span should be specified. Quantitative data is best obtained contemporaneously. How data was recorded is also important. Bluff and Holloway (1994) tape-recorded interviews, but observations may be video-recorded. The impact of each of these needs to be considered in relation to the research findings.

The way in which quantitative as well as qualitative researchers communicate, verbally and nonverbally, may influence participants and the data they collect. The researcher(s) should therefore verbalize any effect they think they might have had. They should also indicate whether they were familiar with the context in which the study took place. You might find this included in a discussion of limitations of the study. The process of discovery particularly associated with qualitative research may be inhibited if the midwife researcher has worked in the setting for a number of years. Familiarity with the setting may lead to assumptions being made that are then inappropriately integrated into the study. If a reflective diary has been kept the researcher will be able to identify how such problems have been minimized. This type of diary has been associated with qualitative researchers but you could also question the need for quantitative researchers to keep a diary.

Data analysis

Quantitative researchers gather data in the form of statistics while qualitative researchers collect data in the form of words. Data analysis is therefore dependent on the approach adopted. Statistical analysis was discussed in Chapter 5. You will need to consider whether the statistics are descriptive or inferential. If the latter, the statistics that have been used will also need to be considered. Most midwives will need to have a good statistical reference book available. It is not necessary to be able to undertake statistical calculations but it is essential that the presence of 'p values', levels of significance, confidence intervals and, increasingly, odds ratios, if presented, are identified and understood. As most papers do not present all the raw data and most practitioners could not recalculate the statistics, the midwife reading any research paper should consider whether there was a statistician in the list of authors, which would increase the validity and reliability of the statistical analysis. You also need to check whether statistical advice was obtained as part of the research design. Some journals undertake a statistical review of quantitative papers; while such a review is not yet universal practice, reputable journals are moving towards this, which allows practitioners to have greater confidence in the information presented. The researcher should make it clear which statistics packages have been used to assist them in analysis of the data as there are small variations between packages.

Analysis of qualitative research data provides an understanding of the phenomenon that was explored. Analysis of data collected using the main approaches has been discussed in Chapters 6, 7 and 8. You would expect the underlying principles of these approaches to have been followed. However, in adapting an approach for the purposes of exploring a particular phenomenon, the researcher(s) should provide a clear explanation or audit trail (Lincoln and

Guba 1985) that makes explicit the process the researcher(s) followed in order to achieve their understanding. A number of features are common to all qualitative approaches. Interviews and observations are transcribed. Who did the transcribing should be stipulated in the text. Transcripts are frequently read or tapes listened to and comparisons made. Recurring themes and patterns are identified by coding or naming the data to give it meaning. Look for examples of some codes, as this can help you to recognize how those with similar meanings have been linked together to form themes or categories. If grounded theory has been used there should be evidence of a core category or story line (Strauss and Corbin 1998). Computer packages such as Ethnograph and Atlas are available to assist qualitative researchers.

FINDINGS, DISCUSSION AND IMPLICATIONS FOR PRACTICE

These three aspects are usually integrated in a qualitative study. In quantitative studies they tend to be considered separately. The findings are the presentation of results of the study. In quantitative studies these should include some raw data, although this will be restricted in a journal article. Tables and graphs are often used to display quantitative data. For example, Cluett et al (1995) used a variety of tables and line and point graphs to display raw data and the analysis based on that data. Care should be taken to ensure that information presented in this way is consistent with statements within the text. Look for results that may not be mentioned but give cause for concern. Thomson (1993) provides one table illustrating the range of neonatal cord pH as 6.9–7. In a small sample of low-risk women even one pH recording of 6.9 is clearly outside the parameter of normality and should be discussed. In experimental research the hypothesis should be accepted or rejected. If other approaches to research were adopted, look to see if aims or objectives were achieved.

A number of phrases in the text may help you to identify the reliance authors place on their findings and the possible significance of those findings for your own practice:

- ✦ it was demonstrated…
- ✦ important findings were…
- ✦ it is recommended that….

Broadly interpreted, these phrases suggest that the research findings were significant and you should consider if they apply to, or could be part of your practice. Other phrases include:

- ✦ data from this study suggest…
- ✦ the study might indicate that…

◆ one conclusion might be...
◆ it could be argued that....

These suggest that the researchers found some interesting outcomes that need further consideration, possibly further studies with larger samples or more specific analysis. This may be because only one perspective has been presented in the article and there may be other findings or perspectives that have yet to be reported or discovered.

Unexpected findings should be mentioned and whether these came from primary or secondary analysis. Incomplete findings should be identified and these, together with the unexpected or those resulting from secondary analysis, often become the suggestions for future research. In their discussion of the findings, quantitative researchers include identification of the strengths and limitations of the study, difficulties encountered and interesting side issues, with reference to other relevant literature.

In qualitative studies there should be evidence to show that the literature has been incorporated into the findings. For this reason, findings and discussion are presented together. The discussion highlights examples from the literature that both support and refute the findings. When comparing and contrasting the literature you may find it helpful to remind yourself of the context in which the study took place.

The use of quotes clearly distinguishes qualitative from quantitative research. They are usually easy to read, give 'life' to the story and should provide support for the researcher's interpretation of the data. You should be able to identify whether the study is descriptive or whether, in the case of a grounded theory study, there is a theory to explain the phenomenon. Illustrations in the form of diagrams may be used. Beck (1993) clearly demonstrates how codes derived from her data analysis were reduced to form categories. As in quantitative research, these should correspond to the written text.

Validity and reliability

Issues of validity and reliability have been considered in Chapters 3 and 4 and have been referred to under data collection. When critiquing the literature it is advisable to consider these issues separately, looking at the complete research design as well as the various components within it.

Trustworthiness of the data

The terms validity and reliability are considered inappropriate for application to qualitative research (Leininger 1985). Hutchinson (1986) notes that quantitative researchers tend to view qualitative research as less rigorous than quantitative research because the reality of how individuals view their world is subjective, as is the researchers' interpretation. Qualitative researchers are, however, equally concerned to ensure the 'truth' or trustworthiness of their data. Researchers should reveal how they came to know they had the truth. Look for an audit trail and member checks (Lincoln and Guba 1985). Do you as the reader recognize the experience? Identify whether saturation of codes and categories has been achieved (Glaser and Strauss 1967, Strauss and Corbin 1998). Findings cannot be generalized to a whole population but you can question whether with a similar sample in a similar environment there is 'transferability' of findings (Lincoln and Guba 1985). Morse (1992) believes that it is possible to generalize some results when existing literature provides evidence of similar findings. This usually applies to abstract concepts. For example, 'fitting in', a central theme in an ongoing study that explores midwives as role models for students (Bluff, ongoing study), can be applicable to numerous situations.

ETHICAL ISSUES

The discussion of ethical issues may be restricted to one section of the study. This may, however, appear disjointed as there is an ethical component at all stages of the research process. Alternatively, the issues may be discussed under each heading in the process. For example, under the heading entitled 'method', whether it is ethical to recruit women to a study when they are particularly vulnerable, such as when they are in labour, and the nature of informed consent may be discussed.

Look to see if the researchers sought permission from the local Ethics Committee to undertake the study. Any research study that samples the women we care for must be submitted to a committee. These committees have a responsibility to peruse the research proposal to ensure that subjects or participants are protected from harm. There should be evidence to show that the researchers gained permission to access the site. Informed consent should be obtained. In quantitative research this is clear-cut but in qualitative research it does create a dilemma. The direction of the study may change as important issues emerge. Look to see what the researcher gained consent for. It is important that researchers aim to be as honest and accurate as possible (Couchman and Dawson 1995).

Confidentiality and anonymity are sometimes used synonymously but are two separate issues. You will need to identify how these were achieved. Particularly consider storage of tapes and video recordings of observations. Pseudonyms should be used in qualitative research, but small sample sizes make the issue of anonymity even more pertinent.

If nonparticipant observation is chosen as a means of collecting data the researcher should have no involvement in the events that are being observed. This is an ethical issue, because if the researcher responds it may influence what events occur next and thus influence the data that is collected. The researcher should make clear the criteria for intervening and if and when s/he did so.

Conclusions

Conclusions should be clear and concise and derived from the findings of the study. You must use your own professional judgement to decide whether you agree with them. Findings are not always conclusive, in which case only suggestions can be made in light of the available evidence. You would therefore expect further research to be recommended.

Implications and recommendations for practice

Recommendations for future practice should reflect the findings and discussion. If research findings are to be applied to your practice you should have judged the research method to be well designed and appropriate for the phenomenon that was studied. Remember, the study should be critiqued with reference to other literature on the topic. Only in this way can a decision be made to either implement findings into your practice or reject them. In quantitative research you will particularly need to be sure that the client group selected has the same characteristics as those where you practise. The issues of transferability or generalizability in qualitative research have already been considered. Researchers who are midwives can discuss implications and make recommendations for future practice. If, however, the researchers are not midwives they will not be in a position to do this and will leave it to you. Implications and recommendations apply to the women, fetus/neonate, their families, midwives and other health professionals as well as provision of the service, which may have cost implications.

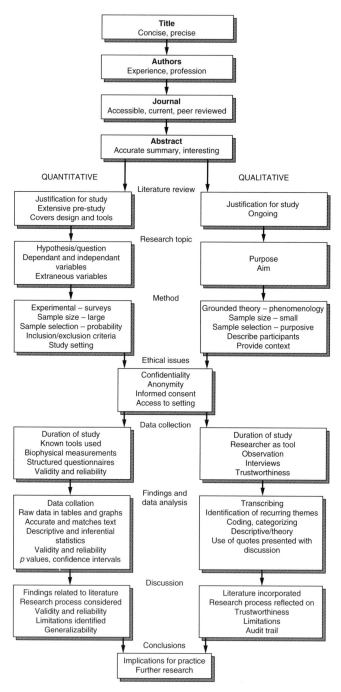

Figure 10.1 Flow chart summarizing the main points to consider when critiquing a research paper

CONCLUSION

It is important that all midwives should keep up to date, which implies reading current literature. This reading should include evaluating the quality of the literature as well as its implications for practice. Critiquing is a skill that develops over time, so select an article on a topic of interest to you and start critiquing. Remember, your clinical experience is valid, so trust your own instincts. If the study seems muddled or unclear it probably is. Instead of a summary box we conclude this chapter with a flow diagram (Fig. 10.1) that summarizes the key points that could be considered as part of your critiquing process. It should not be followed rigidly but considered as a guide to be adapted to meet your needs and modified in the light of the type of article or paper being reviewed.

REFERENCES

Arber S 1993 The research process. In: Gilbert N (ed) Researching social life. Sage Publications, London, ch 3, p 32–51

Beck C T 1993 Teetering on the edge: a substantive theory of postpartum depression. Nursing Research 42(1): 42–48

Bluff R Ongoing study. Fitting in and staying out of trouble: the influence of midwives on student learning. Ongoing research

Bluff R, Holloway I 1994 'They know best': women's perceptions of midwifery care during labour and childbirth. Midwifery 10(3): 157–164

Cluett E R, Alexander J, Pickering R M 1995 Is measuring postnatal symphysis–fundal distance worthwhile? Midwifery 11(4): 174–183

Couchman W, Dawson J 1995 Nursing and health-care research. Scutari Press, London

Cox J L, Holden J, Sagovsky R 1987 Detection of postnatal depression: development of the 10-item Edinburgh Postnatal Depression Scale (EPDS). British Journal of Psychiatry 150: 782–786

Davies R M 1996 'Practitioners in their own right': an ethnographic study of the perceptions of student midwives. In: Robinson S, Thomson A M (ed) Midwives, research and childbirth, vol 4. Chapman & Hall, London, ch 5, p 85–107

De Jong P R, Johanson R B, Baxen P et al 1997 Randomized trial comparing the upright and supine positions for the second stage of labour. British Journal of Obstetrics and Gynaecology 104(5): 567–571

Denzin N 1978 The research act. McGraw-Hill, New York

Glaser B, Strauss A L 1967 The discovery of grounded theory strategies for qualitative research. Aldine Press, Chicago, IL

Grant J M 1995 Randomized trials and the *British Journal of Obstetrics and Gynaecology* minimum requirements for publication. British Journal of Obstetrics and Gynaecology 102(11): 849–850

Holloway I, Wheeler S 1996 Qualitative research for nurses. Blackwell Scientific, Oxford

Hutchinson S 1986 Grounded theory: the method. In: Munhall P L, Oiler C J (ed) Nursing research: a qualitative perspective. Appleton-Century-Crofts, Norwalk, CT, ch 6, p 111–130

Leininger M 1994 Evaluation criteria and critique of qualitative research studies. In: Morse J M (ed) Critical issues in qualitative research methods. Sage Publications, Thousand Oaks, CA, ch 6, p 95–115

Leininger M 1985 Qualitative research methods in nursing. Grune & Stratton, Orlando, FL

Lincoln Y S, Guba E G 1985 Naturalistic inquiry. Sage Publications, Newbury Park, CA

Morse J M 1991 Strategies for sampling. In: Morse J M (ed) Qualitative nursing research a contemporary dialogue. Sage Publications, Newbury Park, CA, ch 8, p 127–145

Morse J M 1992 The power of induction. Qualitative Health Research 2: 3–6

Parahoo K 1997 Nursing research: principles, process and issues. Macmillan, Basingstoke

Paterson J A, Davis J, Gregory M et al 1994 A study of the effects of low haemoglobin on postnatal women. Midwifery 10(2): 77–86

Pocock S J 1983 Clinical trials: a practical approach. John Wiley, Chichester

Polit D F, Hungler B P 1997 Nursing research principles and methods. JB Lippincott, Philadelphia, PA

Price A, Price B 1996 Critical reading. Modern Midwife 7(5): 26–29

Rees C 1994 Evaluating a research article. British Journal of Midwifery 2(12): 596–601

Sandall J 1997 Midwives' burnout and continuity of care. British Journal of Midwifery 5(2): 106–111

Strauss A L, Corbin J 1998 Basics of qualitative research techniques and procedures for developing grounded theory. Sage Publications, Thousand Oaks, CA

Thomson A M 1993 Pushing techniques in the second stage of labour. Journal of Advanced Nursing 18(1): 171–177

From research to practice

Rosalind Bluff   Elizabeth Cluett

KEY ISSUES

◆ Dissemination of research information

◆ Evidence-based practice

◆ Traditional practice

◆ The new midwifery practitioner

◆ Research as a strategy for change

INTRODUCTION

We began this book by highlighting how research is derived from practice. Now we will complete the circle by considering how research findings can be incorporated into clinical practice. The aim of midwifery research is to improve the quality of care offered to mothers and babies. There is therefore little point in midwives and others undertaking research unless the findings are used to influence practice.

This book has explored the quantitative and qualitative research paradigms and the different approaches within these that can be adopted. These have been placed on a continuum according to their characteristics. Some midwives will want to undertake research studies. This book should provide them with a basic knowledge of the research process to help them on their way but they should seek research support. It would, however be inappropriate for all midwives to undertake research and not all would want to do so. Nevertheless, all midwives are required to base their practice on research findings (Department of Health 1993a). This means that midwives and others who undertake research have a responsibility to complete the final stage of the research process by disseminating their findings.

DISSEMINATION OF INFORMATION

Many midwives present their findings at local and national study days as their colleagues believe they should do (Robinson et al 1988). Researchers can also disseminate their findings by submitting them for publication in journals. Many midwives, however, do not do so (Hicks 1993) and the deterrent may be midwives themselves, who do not value research undertaken by their own peers (Hicks 1992).

Researchers should aim to write their work in a way that will be understood. Some midwives perceive that too much jargon is used, which is difficult to interpret (Robinson et al 1988, Meah et al 1996) and data presented in the form of statistics is often difficult to understand (Meah et al 1996). Theses are large and may be difficult to obtain, but articles derived from one study may appear in different journals that take into account different levels of understanding. More research terminology may be found in a journal like *Midwifery*, where there is an assumption that midwives who read it have considerable knowledge of the research process. You may find the *British Journal of Midwifery, Midwives, Practising Midwife* and the *Nursing Times* easier to read until your understanding of the research process increases. Nevertheless, you do have a responsibility to develop a basic level of research knowledge. If you have read part, or all, of this book, you will have enhanced your knowledge and understanding of the research process. You will, however, need to extend your reading, particularly if you are planning to undertake any research project. Chapter 3 provides only an introduction to help you develop this skill.

Those who work in the clinical setting have an equal responsibility to be receptive to researchers' findings. Hicks (1994) points out that, if research findings are to influence practice, midwives must be able to evaluate them. Many midwives do, however, lack the skills to do this (Milne and Hundley 1998). This is also supported by the findings of Harris (1992), who identified that even when research findings were implemented into practice only rarely was it done appropriately. In Chapter 10 we provided guidelines to help you effectively critique the literature so that you can use the evidence to make decisions about care if it is appropriate to do so. With practice you will become skilled at doing this. In this way, research will be influential in ensuring you provide women with a high standard of care. You may find it helpful to undertake an educational programme that enables you to participate with others in developing this skill.

Study days for staff can significantly influence your confidence and ability to interpret the literature, with the potential for findings to be incorporated into practice (Hicks 1994). Some midwives have expressed concern that they are not supported by their managers, who expect them to pay their own fees and use their days off to attend (Meah et al 1996). You may need to be proactive in identifying ways in which you can gain access to the literature and develop the skills you need. Staffing levels and workload may mean a commitment to using some of your own time to do this. You must demonstrate that you have updated yourself on issues relevant to your practice setting to meet the requirements for professional relicensing (UKCC 1994), but you do not have to attend study days to do this. You could, for example, negotiate to spend time in the library doing your own literature review on an issue relevant to your practice. Some midwives have done this for you in the Alexander et al series of Research Based Practice books. The Royal College of Midwives, in their guide to breastfeeding (Royal College of Midwives 1991), also provides a comprehensive review of the literature designed to ensure that midwives give women consistent information to support them with breastfeeding. These initiatives have made it easier for midwives to access information.

Parker (1994) has suggested that midwives may not read journals relevant to their practice. Journals can have an influence on clinical practice. Smith (1996) believes that this is based on the contribution they make to the development of the individual practitioner, the profession and the advancement of the body of knowledge. The journals mentioned above are all available to midwives via library facilities or personal subscriptions. You might argue that they are expensive, but you could get together with two or three other midwives and share the journals you subscribe to. Milne and Hundley (1998) suggest establishing a journal club or discussion group. In this way you can be proactive in discussing articles with your colleagues and undertake joint critiquing, helping each other to develop the skills you need. Articles from consumer journals could also be reviewed as much can be learned from our clients' perspective of the factors that affect their lives and the care we offer. Midwives must be equipped to give care that is based on knowledge of these many factors. Page (1998) acknowledges the influence of the media in disseminating information to women. When this information is inaccurate it is important that midwives have the knowledge to counteract the adverse effects this may have by providing a balanced view.

The Midwives Information and Resource Service (MIDIRS) regularly publishes a *Midwifery Digest* containing articles, abstracts and summaries derived from literature relevant to midwifery. This information is also available on a database. The Cochrane Database of Pregnancy and Childbirth makes current evidence on effective and safe maternity care available to all practitioners. *A Guide to Effective Care in Pregnancy and Childbirth*, published in paperback (Enkin et al 1995), is an effective means of providing in easy-to-read form what is on the database. This is not, however, as up to date as the database, which is updated quarterly. Remember, it is a systematic review of randomized control trials, although conclusions are considered with reference to other types of research. Other databases include Medline, Sociofile, Psyclit, CINHAL and the Internet's World Wide Web.

MIDIRS provides an enquiry service and on request will do searches for you on its database. Nevertheless, you need to develop your skills in technology so you can find your own evidence. In the future it is likely that there will be computer programmes available for you to access in your clinical setting. Midwives can experience anxiety associated with a lack of computer skills to enable them to access databases (Meah et al 1996). You may want to investigate whether the initiative established by Littler and Weist (1998), which involved providing the educational support to familarize staff with ward-based access to computer databases, can be done in your unit.

Gaining access to information is not always easy. Inevitably, knowledge of research findings is limited when access to that knowledge is limited (Meah et al 1996). Mergers of schools of midwifery with schools of nursing and subsequently with universities means that library facilities may not be on your work site. Lack of time 'to access information' (Milne and Hundley 1998) and time 'to reflect' (Hurley 1998) and charges for using the facilities may prevent you from accessing information (Milne and Hundley 1998). Remember, learning is a two-way process and midwives can help each other. You can also learn from students. Our own experience suggests that students want you to facilitate their learning in the clinical setting. Students also want to share their knowledge and discuss why certain care is given, particularly when that care is not based on evidence they know is available. This means you have to be prepared for your practice to be challenged and this is not always comfortable. You are in effect being told that the care you have been giving to women is incorrect. However, we act on the basis of the knowledge we have at the time. Remember that knowledge is changing and you can avoid the discomfort by keeping up to date yourself. Importantly, be receptive and open-minded rather than acting defensively.

EVIDENCE-BASED PRACTICE

Clinical governance focuses on achieving clinical effectiveness and quality of care in the health services (Department of Health 1998b). A key component of this is evidence-based practice. As a midwife you are accountable for your own practice (UKCC 1992, 1998) and must act always in the best interests of clients (UKCC 1992). Research identifies what is or is not safe practice. A major influence on the quality of care women receive is therefore the ability of midwives to use their knowledge of research findings to make appropriate decisions. The Department of Health (1996) provides a classification for the evidence that practitioners can use to inform their practice. This places research findings based on randomized control trials at the top of a hierarchy, followed by other experimental studies. Qualitative research findings are not considered as evidence. You may not find this surprising when you consider that doctors have long been recognized as having the position of power in the hospital hierarchy (Freidson 1975) and until recently have placed little value on qualitative research findings. You will, however, need to use qualitative research findings to make decisions if you are to provide holistic and individualized care that takes into account the social, psychological, emotional, spiritual and educational needs of women as well as their physical needs.

We now know women want choice and control of the care they receive (Department of Health 1993a). The Department of Health (1993a) advocates that health professionals involved in maternity care should work in partnership with clients in order to achieve this. Through sharing knowledge of research findings, midwives can provide women with options of care so they are empowered to make informed decisions based on reliable evidence. In this way women can act as their own advocates. This process has been facilitated by MIDIRS, in conjunction with the NHS Centre for Reviews and Dissemination, which has so far produced 10 Informed Choice leaflets for both women and professionals on such issues as support in labour (MIDIRS 1996a, 1996b), ultrasound (MIDIRS 1996c, 1996d), antenatal screening for congenital abnormalities (MIDIRS 1997a, 1997b), and breast- and bottle-feeding (MIDIRS 1997c, 1997d). It is important that midwives are aware of these leaflets and that a version of each leaflet written in lay language is also published for clients. These leaflets also inform women that they can ask for the professional's version. They are not, however, universally available.

Organizations representing clients are committed to ensuring that maternity care is based on research evidence. The National Childbirth Trust, with the help of its Research and Information Group, aims to identify inappropriate practices, review the literature and distribute accurate up-to-date information on these practices, not only to their own members but also to those professionals involved in the provision of maternity services and to other pressure groups (Gyte 1994). According to Gyte (1994), success in producing and disseminating this information is dependent on collaboration.

Midwives need to be aware that these initiatives mean that many pregnant women have knowledge corresponding to their own, and you should be prepared to be challenged about the care you offer if it does not correspond to the information available to women. You will also need to consider the effect this may have on your relationship with clients. The application of the medical model of care has resulted in what Szasz and Hollender (1956) call the active passivity relationship, in which clients are the passive recipients of care. This is not the partnership the *Changing Childbirth* report (Department of Health 1993a) refers to. If clients have the information to make their own informed decisions with your help, your relationship will change to one of mutual participation, as described by Szasz and Hollender (1956). You will, however, need to be flexible. Some women may want you to make decisions for them. Raphael-Leff (1991) describes the characteristics of women, whom she calls 'regulators', who want health practitioners to be in control of their care. It should, however, be the clients' choice that the midwife makes decisions for them and not an assumption that we make. The change in maternity care culture means that paternalism is no longer acceptable. Even if women want to make decisions they may still need midwives to be their advocates, particularly in labour when in pain, tired or drugged. It can be difficult even for the most assertive woman to be her own advocate in these situations. Remember, women trust midwives and believe they know what care is best for them (Bluff and Holloway 1994). The decisions you make should, therefore, be based wherever possible on research findings, otherwise you will be abusing this trust. Occasionally, clients may reject research-based evidence or inappropriately use it to support their own wishes. Or you may not be happy with the decisions they make. Legally you will, however, still be required to provide midwifery care. Your Supervisor of Midwives is available to discuss professional issues with you and the whole issue of supervision has recently been researched (Kirkham 1996).

Research evidence can be used to assist in the development of guidelines for practice (Department of Health 1993b). This can extend to policies. According to Milne and Hundley (1998), these should not only be based on up-to-date research findings but also reflect the woman as the focus of care, and be reviewed to ensure they continue to be based on appropriate evidence. The integration of woman-centred care can be likened to combining the art and science in midwifery.

The Department of Health (1993b) recommends that standards of care specified in contracts between purchasers and providers of health care should be based on evidence. In this way the quality of care clients will receive can be made explicit. Midwives have a major responsibility in ensuring these standards are maintained by using evidence to support their practice, and therefore have an influence on whether these contracts are renewed.

Clinical practice should be regularly audited (Department of Health 1993a, 1993b) and this is another feature of clinical governance (Department of Health 1998b) that will need to be undertaken by midwives. Auditing can promote excellence in practice by identifying whether we integrate up to date evidence into our practice (Hundley and Graham 1997). For example, the literature might suggest that a particular type of suture material is most effective for repairing the perineum following childbirth. If this is not being used in your unit an audit can be undertaken to confirm what suture material is used. Outcomes such as perineal infection, wound breakdown, perineal pain and discomfort can be compared with those of the recommended suture material. In this way the benefits of the recommended material can be compared with those you use. If it is identified that the research evidence is not incorporated into practice there should be a commitment to change practice.

TRADITIONAL PRACTICE

So far we have considered how research can both enhance the midwife's practice and the care that mothers and babies receive. Despite recognition of the need to incorporate research findings into clinical practice, Harris (1992), Department of Health (1993a), Hicks (1994) and Hurley (1998) acknowledge that some midwifery practices are still based on traditional knowledge. A number of reasons may account for this. Research evidence is not always available to support your practice. Sometimes results are not conclusive but suggestions may be made, which you will have to take into consideration when giving care. Flaws in design or inappropriate conclusions may sometimes mean the evidence is unreliable. There may also be occasions when you have to reserve judgement about the value of a piece of research until further evidence confirms or refutes the findings. In these situations you will have to make decisions based on other sources of knowledge. Those decisions can be enhanced by an understanding of epistemology or the theory of knowledge, in other words where that knowledge comes from, what is or is not an appropriate source of knowledge and how that knowledge is used. Types of knowledge that the midwife relies on were considered in Chapter 2.

You may feel, as Hicks (1994) suggests, that you lack the autonomy necessary to provide care based on evidence. The hospital environment is particularly noted for policies that inform the midwife's practice. These tend to reflect the medical model of care. Doctors have been a major influence in formulating them (Garcia and Garforth 1989) and they are known to restrict the midwife's practice (Robinson et al 1983, Bluff, ongoing study). Not all, however, have been updated to reflect current knowledge. Some midwives have a negative attitude towards research and its influence on practice (Hicks 1993) and may adversely affect midwives who are favourably disposed to implementing research findings. Bluff (ongoing study) found that, despite a legal responsibility to maintain and update their own professional practice (UKCC 1998), midwives she labelled 'prescriptive' did not meet this requirement and continued to base their practice on traditional knowledge. The expectation that other midwives would practise in a similar way resulted in intimidation, which inhibited some midwives from integrating research findings into their practice.

THE NEW PRACTITIONER

Midwives who use research findings and other evidence to make decisions use their professional judgement to provide appropriate care. In this way, they are able to justify their practice and act autonomously, rather than relying on doctors to make decisions for them. The UKCC (1986) emphasized this autonomy and the practitioner as a 'knowledgeable doer' when they referred to the 'new' practitioner who would emerge as a result of a new philosophy and approach to educational programmes. Research findings, in adding to the professional body of knowledge, can also enhance the midwife's ability to communicate at the same level as doctors, so that they can more effectively collaborate in care as they are required to do (UKCC 1992). In this way, if it is appropriate, midwives can act as advocates for women. You can also be flexible, because you know what options are available, and can adjust care according to the individual needs of clients. Your knowledge of the evidence will also challenge you to think and question the care you and other health professionals give. This can increase your confidence and ability to be assertive and enhance your job satisfaction. Reflection 'on' and 'in' action (Schön 1987) will enhance your ability to learn from experience and enable this learning to be compared with what you gain through reading and critiquing the literature.

RESEARCH AS A STRATEGY FOR CHANGE

The recommendations of the Department of Health (1993a) provide midwives

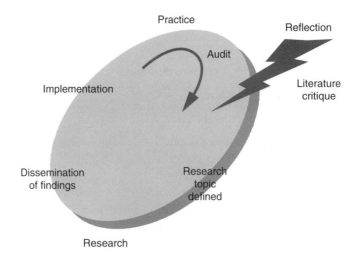

Figure 11.1 A strategy for change

with the opportunity to fulfil the scope of the midwife's role and be autonomous practitioners. Rowan and Steele (1995) acknowledge that this is an opportunity to change attitudes, practice and behaviour. Figure 11.1 provides a strategy for change which completes the practice to research cycle.

It is one thing to change your own practice but to influence and change the practice of others can be very difficult to achieve. You will need to act as a change agent and success may well depend on a knowledge of change theory and possession of good interpersonal skills. Harris (1992) acknowledges the need for midwives to have the support of managers and educators if they are to implement research findings. If you feel you lack this support it does not mean that you cannot incorporate research findings into your practice. In your own practice you will interact with the women you care for. You can share the information you have and provide them with opportunities to make their own decisions. In this way you can set an example for others by acting as a positive role model.

CONCLUSION

If research findings are to be implemented into practice midwives need access to the literature and skills to critique the research evidence and implement strategies for change. The culture of midwifery is changing and midwives can help and support each other in undertaking research or being research-aware. 'The integration of midwifery research and practice should be nurtured' (Department of Health 1998a, p. 4). In this way, midwives can ensure that all women receive quality care that is based on sound evidence.

CHAPTER SUMMARY

- ◆ Midwives who undertake research have a responsibility to disseminate their findings
- ◆ Practice based on traditional knowledge is no longer acceptable
- ◆ All midwives have a responsibility to use research findings as evidence on which to base their practice, when it is appropriate to do so
- ◆ To promote quality midwifery care, current research findings should be used to formulate policies and guidelines that inform practice
- ◆ Midwives and students can help and support each other in the provision of care by sharing their knowledge
- ◆ Research can be likened to a circle that begins when questions are generated from clinical practice. The circle is completed when findings are incorporated into practice.

REFERENCES

Bluff R, Holloway I 1994 'They know best': women's perceptions of midwifery care during labour and childbirth. Midwifery 10(3): 157–164

Bluff R (ongoing study) Fitting in and staying out of trouble: The influence of midwives on student learning.

Department of Health 1993a Report of the Expert Maternity Group: changing childbirth. HMSO, London

Department of Health 1993b Research for health. Department of Health, London

Department of Health 1996 Promoting clinical effectiveness: a framework for action in and through the NHS. National Health Service Executive, Leeds

Department of Health 1998a Midwifery: delivering our future. Report by the Standing Nursing and Midwifery Advisory Committee. Department of Health, London

Department of Health 1998b Clinical governance: key points. Press release 98/141. Department of Health, London

Enkin M, Keirse M J N C, Renfrew M, Neilson J 1995 A guide to effective care in pregnancy and childbirth. Oxford University Press, Oxford

Freidson E 1975 Profession of medicine: a study of the sociology of applied knowledge. Dodd, Mead & Co, New York

Garcia J, Garforth S 1989 Labour and delivery routines in English consultant units. Midwifery 5: 155–162

Gyte G 1994 Putting research into practice in maternity care. Modern Midwife 4(8): 19–20

Harris M 1992 The impact of research findings on current practice in relieving postpartum perineal pain in a large district general hospital. Midwifery 8(3): 125–131

Hicks C 1992 Research in midwifery: are midwives their own worst enemies? Midwifery 8(1): 12–18

Hicks C 1993 A survey of midwives' attitudes to, and involvement in research: the first stage in identifying the needs for a staff development programme. Midwifery 9: 51–62

Hicks C 1994 Bridging the gap between research and practice: an assessment of the value of a study day in developing critical reading skills in midwives. Midwifery 10(1): 18–25

Hundley V, Graham W 1997 Research and audit in midwifery: does the difference matter? British Journal of Midwifery 5(11): 664–668

Hurley J 1998 Midwives and research-based practice. British Journal of Midwifery 6(5): 294–297

Kirkham M (editor) 1996 Supervision of midwives. Books for Midwives Press, Cheshire

Littler C, Weist A 1998 Front-line evidence-based midwifery. Midwives 1(9): 282–284

Meah S, Luke K A, Cullum N A 1996 An exploration of midwives' attitudes to research and perceived barriers to research utilization. Midwifery 12(2): 73–84

MIDIRS/NHS Centre for Reviews and Dissemination 1996a Support in labour. Informed choice for women. Midwives' Information and Research Service, Bristol

MIDIRS/NHS Centre for Reviews and Dissemination 1996b Support in labour. Informed choice for professionals. Midwives' Information and Research Service, Bristol

MIDIRS/NHS Centre for Reviews and Dissemination 1996c Ultrasound scans: should you have one? Informed choice for women. Midwives' Information and Research Service, Bristol

MIDIRS/NHS Centre for Reviews and Dissemination 1996d Ultrasound screenings in the first half of pregnancy: is it useful for everyone? Informed choice for professionals. Midwives' Information and Research Service, Bristol

MIDIRS/NHS Centre for Reviews and Dissemination 1997a Looking for Down's syndrome and spina bifida in pregnancy. Informed choice for women. Midwives' Information and Research Service, Bristol

MIDIRS/NHS Centre for Reviews and Dissemination 1997b Antenatal screening for congenital abnormalities: helping women to choose. Informed choice for professionals. Midwives' Information and Research Service, Bristol

MIDIRS/NHS Centre for Reviews and Dissemination 1997c Feeding your baby – breast or bottle? Informed choice for women. Midwives' Information and Research Service, Bristol

MIDIRS/NHS Centre for Reviews and Dissemination 1997d Breastfeeding or bottle feeding: helping women to choose. Informed choice for professionals. Midwives' Information and Research Service, Bristol

Milne J, Hundley V 1998 A strategy for raising research awareness among midwives. British Journal of Midwifery 6(6): 374–375

Page L 1998 Evidence based practice – or trial by newspaper. British Journal of Midwifery 6(8): 497

Parker C 1994 Breastfeeding: research and quality assurance issues. Midwifery, British Journal of Midwifery 2(2): 56–60

Raphael-Leff J 1991 The psychological process of childbirth. Chapman & Hall, London

Robinson S, Golden J, Bradley S 1983 A study of the role and responsibilities of the midwife. NERU Report no 1. Nursing Education Research Unit, King's College, London

Robinson S, Thomson A, Tickner V 1988 Midwives' views on directions and developments in midwifery research. In: Robinson S, Thomson A, Tickner V (ed) Research and the Midwife Conference proceedings for 1988. Department of Nursing, University of Manchester, Manchester

Rowan M, Steele R 1995 Effective change through vision, attitude, reflection and innovation. In: 'Changing childbirth': an educational resource for midwives. Section 5: The challenge of change. English National Board, London, p 8–20

Royal College of Midwives 1991 Successful breast feeding, 2nd edn. Royal College of Midwives in conjunction with Churchill Livingstone, London

Schön D A 1987 Educating the reflective practitioner. Jossey-Bass, San Francisco, CA

Smith J P 1996 The role of nursing journals in the advancement of professional nursing. Journal of Advanced Nursing 23(1): 12–16

Szasz T S, Hollender M H 1956 A contribution to the philosophy of medicine. The basic models of the doctor patient relationship. Archives of Internal Medicine 97: 585–592

UKCC 1986 Project 2000: a new preparation for practice. United Kingdom Central Council for Nursing, Midwifery and Health Visiting, London

UKCC 1992 Code of professional conduct. United Kingdom Central Council for Nursing, Midwifery and Health Visiting, London

UKCC 1994 The future of professional practice. The council's standards for education and practice following registration. United Kingdom Central Council for Nursing, Midwifery and Health Visiting, London

UKCC 1998 Midwives' rules and code of practice. United Kingdom Central Council for Nursing, Midwifery and Health Visiting, London

Glossary

Absolute risk reduction   A percentage that indicates how many individuals fewer there will be with the complication/disorder if they receive the experimental treatment/management compared to if they had received the control or standard option

Abstract   A brief summary of a research study

Action research   Research that aims to implement and evaluate changes in practice

Analysis   Methods of organizing and understanding data

Analysis of variance or ANOVA   A procedure that considers the significance of the difference between the means of the groups in an experimental study, using the variance as the indicator of this difference, when there are three or more groups being studied

Anthropology   The study of people within their culture; the discipline from which ethnography is derived

Audit trail   The means by which each step of the qualitative research process is made explicit

Axial coding   A process associated with grounded theory that enables categories to be linked together by identifying their relationship with each other

Beneficence   An ethical principle that aims to achieve what is of benefit to the individual

Bias   Any feature that has the potential to skew research or research findings, intentionally or accidentally

Blinding   When the study participants (single blinding) do not know whether they are in the intervention group or the control group; double blinding is when neither the participants or the researchers know the allocation

Block randomization   A randomization process to ensure equal distribution of participants across trial groups

Bracketing   A term used by phenomenologists to mean the suspension of the researcher(s) knowledge and beliefs to avoid influencing the study

Case study   A research approach that explores a single unit such as an individual or institution

Category   A number of codes with similar meaning grouped together

Categorical statistics   Statistical processes and tests applied to data that is classified into categories

Causal   Where the aim is to identify whether the relationship between the variables under study is causal, i.e. A causes B; this is achieved through experimental studies

Central tendency   Measures that identify the middle or average of the group; these are the mean, median and mode

Code   A word or words used during the process of analysis that gives meaning to qualitative data

Coding   The process of naming or labelling qualitative data to give it meaning and determine themes and patterns

Concept   An idea, which may be concrete or abstract

Conceptual density   Associated with a theory in which concepts are clearly related to each other and variations in the phenomenon are identified

Concurrent validity   When the validity of a test/measure/tool is shown to be stable in relation to an outside criterion, which is already validated and obtained at approximately the same time as that under consideration

Confidence interval   A descriptive statistic indicating the population parameters for a particular characteristic; it indicates the magnitude of uncertainty associated with the mean value of a sample and gives upper and lower limits, which is a range, between which the population mean is likely to lie, based on the sample's mean and standard deviation

Confirmability   An issue of trustworthiness in which findings of a qualitative study are recognized as a reflection of the research and not the researcher(s) biases

Confounding variable   The same as an extraneous variable, i.e. a variable that is outside the control of the study or is unexpected, but which might impact on the research findings

Constant comparative method   A feature of grounded theory in which each piece of data is frequently compared with all other data collected

Construct validity   The extent to which the test/measurement/tool being used adequately encompasses the construct (i.e. concept or feature) being investigated

Content analysis   A process of quantifying qualitative data

Content validity   A test/measure/tool that encompasses all the required components of the topic under study

Continuous data   The numerical value is continuous, i.e. it can be measured in fractions of the whole, such as in litres or grams

Control group   The group receiving the standard/current/no treatment, used for comparison against the treatment or study group

Convenience sample   The nonprobability selection of the study participation; usually subjects are readily accessible

Core category   The main theme that emerges from the data in a grounded theory study and explains what is happening in the social setting

Correlational   A relationship between the variables under study; for example, as A increases B increases but there is no evidence that A causes B – indeed it is possible that an unknown factor C causes both A and B

Credibility   An issue of trustworthiness in qualitative research: a study is said to have credibility when participants and those familiar with the study topic recognize the findings to be true

Criterion-related validity   A test/measure/tool that provides information compatible with data from another source on the same topic

Crossover design   Where the subjects have a period of 'intervention' and then a period of 'no intervention' and any changes are recorded

Critique   Reviewing a research study to identify its strengths and weaknesses

Data   The information obtained and/or used with any study

Deductive   The process by which a theory is tested

Dependent variable   The outcome measured, or the effect in an experimental study

Descriptive statistics   Statistics that present a picture of the group, i.e. describe the group; these statistics include measures of central tendency and dispersal

Design   The plan of the research, usually related to quantitative research

Deterministic   Where the aim is to determine the presence and magnitude of any relationship between subjects, events, or processes and ultimately to see if there is evidence of cause and effect; linked to experimental research

Dependability   An issue of trustworthiness demonstrated by the ability of another researcher to follow the same qualitative audit trail with similar findings

Discrete data   Numerical data that can only be considered in whole numbers

Donabedian approach   An approach to setting standards that specifies structure, process and outcome

Double hermeneutic   The researcher's interpretation of participants' interpretations of their experiences

Emic perspective   The participants' or 'insiders'' perspective of their own experiences

Epistemology   The study of the nature of knowledge

Ethnography   Research that seeks to explore and understand a culture or group of individuals

Etic perspective   The researcher's interpretations of participants' experiences or behaviour

Evaluation research   An approach to research that focuses on evaluating the effects of practice, decision-making and other issues

Exclusion criteria   Characteristics that make an individual unsuitable for participation in the research study

Existentialist philosophy   Existence through experience

Experimental   A research approach that involves the manipulation of variables, such as in the randomized controlled trial

Ex post facto   Research that is conducted 'after the fact', i.e. using data that is already available

Extraneous variables   Factors that are outside the control of the study, or are unexpected, but might impact the research findings

Factorial design   A design of randomized controlled trial that enables two or more variables to be considered within one study

Feminist research   An approach to research that emphasizes the feminine perspective

Field notes   Written accounts of the researcher's observations and thoughts, completed in the research setting or field as qualitative data is collected

Fieldwork   An ethnographic term that refers to gathering data in a setting

Gate-keepers   Individuals who enable the researcher(s) to gain access to the field or setting for the purpose of undertaking a research study

Generality   A term used when the findings from a qualitative study are considered to be applicable to another similar group

Going native   Adopting the cultural identity of the society or group which is being studied

Grounded theory   An approach to collecting and analysing qualitative data that facilitates the generation of theory both inductively and deductively by constantly comparing one piece of data with another

Hawthorne effect   The change that results from the research process and not the interventions within the research

Hermeneutic philosophy   Concerned with the interpretation of phenomena

Historical research   Research that explores past events

Humanistic   Taking a person-centred approach

Hypothetico-deductive   A hypothetical theory is proposed and then tested

Hypothesis   A statement indicating the suggested relationship between the intervention – the independent variable – and the outcomes – the dependent variables

Inclusion criteria   The characteristics that determine the suitability of individuals for participation in a study

Independent variable   The intervention that is being studied, or the cause in an experimental study

Inductive   Generating theory from the data

Inferential statistics   Statistical processes and tests that aim to provide information that can be used to infer the findings from a study to the general population, or to a similar group in the future

Informants   Members of the sample in qualitative studies

Intersubjectivity   The belief that a shared experience can exist

Inter-rater variability   The amount of agreement achieved/disagreement that occurs when different people undertake the same measurement

Intrarater variability   The degree to which one person obtains the same results when taking the same measurement repeatedly

Interpretist   The qualitative paradigm associated with interpreting/giving meaning to data

Interval data   When the 'distance' or degree of change between the statements on a measurement scale or between numbers is identical

Interquartile range   A measure of dispersal used when the median is the central tendency indicator used, it is the distance between the 25th and the 75th centile

Likert scale   A measurement scale using a series of statements to judge a respondent's attitude to any topic

Lived experience   Perceptions of one's own experience

Manipulation   An intervention, usually instigated or defined by the researchers, the effects of which are under investigation

Matched pairs   Where two subjects are selected to be a pair because of closely matching characteristics

Mean   The arithmetic average obtained by adding the scores of all measurements/items and dividing them by the number of measurements/items

Measures of dispersal   Descriptive statistics that indicate the degree to which the elements are spread out around the central point; these include the range and standard deviation

Median   The midpoint of the data set, when all measurements/items are in numerical order

Memos   Written records of the analytic process used by grounded theorists

Meta-analysis   A research process that involves a systematic review of all the research literature, published and unpublished, that is available on a topic; advanced statistical processes are used to combine the results from the various studies to provide a guide to best practice

Method   The tools and techniques used to undertake a research study, or all the information needed for other researchers to replicate a study

Methodology   The theoretical beliefs, or the perspective on which the study is based

Method slurring   The blurring of research approaches through the combining of methods

Mode   A measure of central tendency; the most popular measurement/item of a data set

Nonexperimental   A research approach or method that does not involve any manipulation of the variables, such as survey research

Nonmaleficence   The principle of doing no harm to individuals

Nonparametric   Statistical tests that can be used when data is categorical in nature or does not meet the criteria for analysis using parametric tests

Nonprobability sample   Where the sample is selected through anything other than a randomization process, for example convenience sample, purposive samples

Nominal data   Data that are ascribed a number as a form of identification when that number has no mathematical value

Normal distribution   Where the distribution of the variable under study can be plotted on a frequency graph and give a symmetrical curve about a central point at which the mean, median and mode all occur

Null hypothesis   A statement indicating that there is no difference in outcomes between participants who received the 'intervention' and the control group

Numbers needed to treat   An indication of the number of individuals who would have to be treated by a new option to prevent an adverse outcome

Numerical data   Where the data is at ratio or interval level and therefore most statistical processes can be applied to it

Objectivity   The attempt to consider the research process, data and analysis from a detached perspective, so data/findings are not influenced by the individual involved in the process

Odds ratio   A summary statistic, defined as the ratio of two odds, which is the comparison of the chances (odds) of subjects with outcome A having been in circumstances Z or not with the chances of subjects not having outcome A, having been in circumstances Z or not

Open sampling Being open to interviewing any participant, observing events or examining any documents that might provide data of interest to the study

Ordinal data Where the 'distance' or degree of change between two adjacent statements or numbers is different to that between other statements or numbers on the same scale

Paradigm A particular perspective or point of view

Parametric test Statistical tests that can be conducted when the data is numerical and fits a normal distribution curve

Participant The individual or subject in a research study

Peer review The review of a research paper by members of your own discipline with appropriate knowledge to assess the quality of the paper prior to publication

Phenomenology A philosophy or research approach that gives meaning to the 'lived' experience of individuals

Phenomenon (*plural* **Phenomena**) The process or concept under consideration

Pilot A trial of the research process on a small scale to test the tools and techniques of the study; may also be used to check feasibility, likely recruitment and outcomes

Population All individuals who could be the subjects of study

Positivist A perspective on research that strives to be scientific, so that it assumes a logical and objective stance; associated with quantitative research

Power calculations The statistical process to calculate the required sample size to achieve statistical significant results in relation to the identified outcome measures of the study

Predictive validity When the test/measure/tool is shown to be stable in comparison with an already validated criteria that is obtained some time in the future

Primary source A research article/paper that is original data

Probability The likelihood of one event occurring compared to the total number of times it is possible for that event to occur

Probability sampling A method of sampling that ensures that all members of the target population have a known chance of being in the study sample

Proposal A description of the research investigation under consideration, including background, research process and proposed analysis methods; usually required when seeking funding or ethical approval

Prospective A study when the data is collected as part of the research process, as opposed to a **retrospective study**, which uses data already available

Proxemics How people use the space which they occupy

Purposive sampling Selecting participants who have knowledge of the topic being studied

Quasi-experimental Where one of the three defining characteristics of an experiment is missing, usually randomization

Qualitative Research that collects data in the form of words and aims to describe and attribute meaning to events and the relationship between them

Quantitative   Where the research aims to collect data that can be analysed numerically and aims to describe and explain events/characteristics, and relationships between events/characteristics, in an objective and numerical manner

Questionnaires   A research tool used to collect data, usually but not exclusively quantitative data

Quota sample   A nonprobability form of sampling where the researchers aim to recruit a specific number of individuals from stated groups and subgroups, with specific characteristics; usually associated with market research and survey methods

Randomization   The allocation of subjects to either the intervention or control group by chance, usually using computer-generated random numbers

Random sample   The same as probability sampling, where every member of the population has a known chance of being selected for the study sample

Range   The distance between the minimum and maximum values of the data

Ratio data   Where the numbers used are progressive, with identical spacing between each number, and there is an absolute zero

Reflexivity   The ability to reflect on the research process and the influence of self on that process

Regression line   A line calculated from correlational studies to enable the prediction of changes in one variable as a second variable changes

Relative risk reduction   A proportion that indicates the difference between the proportion of an experimental group who had a 'condition' and the proportion in the control group who had the 'condition'

Reliability   The consistency with which a tool can measure what it is intended to measure, in the given environment

Retrospective   A study that uses data about events that have already happened

Sample   The group of individuals selected from a target population as representative of that population

Sampling frame   The eligible population from which the sample can be selected

Saturation   When no new ideas emerge from the data in a qualitative study

Selective coding   The process of identifying the core category or story line and relating it to all the other categories

Semistructured interview   A type of interview associated with qualitative research in which open-ended questions are asked that focus on key concepts

Significance   When related to statistics, this is an indicator of the reliability that can be attributed to any results obtained as a measure of the chance/probability that the outcome obtained could be due to chance and not to the feature(s) under investigation

Snowball sampling   A form of purposive sampling that involves one participant recommending the name of another who might be willing to participate in a qualitative study

Standard deviation A measure of dispersal of the subjects around the mean

Standard error The standard deviation that would be obtained if the means from many samples undergoing the same study were obtained; it is calculated from the sample size and the standard deviation of the sample

Statistics Methods used to collate and analyse numerical data

Story line *see* **Core category**

Stratified sample A process to ensure that the composition of the randomly selected research group reflects the composition of the target population in respect to the stratified characteristic, e.g. age or gender

Structured interview A type of interview associated with quantitative research in which questions are presented in the same order and format to each research participant/subject

Study population The group of potential participants that fit the key characteristics for the study

Subject An individual who is participating within a research quantitative study

Survey A nonexperimental, quantitative research approach that aims to collect descriptive or correlational data about a population

Symbolic interactionism A sociological term that focuses on the belief that individuals actively participate or interact with each other and their environment and in doing so actively determine their own behaviour

Systematic review The process by which all the available evidence on one topic is located and evaluated to identify the best possible guide to practice

Systematic sampling Where every nth person from the target population is approached for participation in the research study

Target population sample Every individual in a carefully defined group that meets the inclusion criteria is approached to participate in the research

Theoretical sampling Sampling that is determined by the concepts, categories and emerging theory that is grounded in the data

Theoretical sensitivity The ability of the researcher to give meaning to data collected in a grounded theory study

Thick description A detailed description of a phenomenon and the context in which it is studied

Total population sample Every individual in the group is included

Transferability The ability to transfer qualitative research findings to similar contexts with similar groups

Triangulation The use of a combination of methodologies and/or methods within a methodology to answer a research question

Trustworthiness The extent to which a piece of qualitative research represents the truth – a term used by qualitative researchers in place of **validity** and **reliability**

Type I error An error that occurs when a null hypothesis that is true is rejected

Type II error An error that occurs when a null hypothesis that is false is accepted

Unstructured interview An interview that relies on one or two open-ended questions to obtain qualitative data

Validity   The degree to which a tool/design measures what it is intended to

Variables   Characteristics that are either under study, or controlled for, or occur accidentally but can affect the research findings

Variability   The degree to a which data set is dispersed or spread out

Variance   A measure of dispersal, calculated as part of the standard deviation and used in ANOVA statistical tests

Visual analogue scale   A scale used to measure clinical characteristics such as pain or anxiety where participants are asked to rate the characteristic on a straight line, usually with the best/worse or lowest/highest score being at each extreme of the line

Index

Page numbers in italic refer to glossary entries.

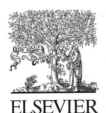

ELSEVIER

 Books *for* **Midwives**

 Mosby 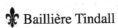 **THE PRACTISING MIDWIFE** **Baillière Tindall**

CHURCHILL LIVINGSTONE

MIDWIFERY PUBLISHERS OF CHOICE FOR GENERATIONS

For many years and through several identities we have catered for professional needs in midwifery education and practice. Leading publishers of major textbooks such as *Myles Textbook for Midwives* and *Mayes' Midwifery: a Textbook for Midwives*, our expertise spreads across both books and journals to offer a comprehensive resource for midwives at all stages of their careers.

Find out how we can provide you with the right book at the right time by exploring our website, **www.elsevierhealth.com/midwifery** or requesting a midwifery catalogue from Health Professions Marketing, Elsevier, 32 Jamestown Road, Camden, London, NW1 7BY, UK Tel: 020 7424 4200; Fax: 202 7424 4420.

We are always keen to expand our midwifery list so if you have an idea for a new book please contact Mary Seager, Senior Commissioning Editor at Elsevier, The Boulevard, Langford Lane, Kidlington, Oxford, OX5 1GB, UK (m.seager@elsevier.com).

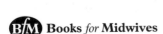 **Have you joined yet?**
Sign up for e-Alert to get the latest news and information.

Register for eAlert at www.elsevierhealth.com/eAlert Information direct to your Inbox

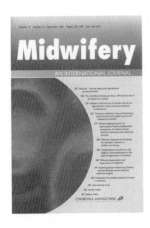

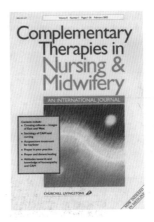